Praise for *The*

"Is there anything more compelling than a life-changing *and* life-saving transformation? In contemporary society, one of the hardest things to do is live your values, embrace your inherent compassion, and be accepted for your authenticity. In *The Vegan Transformation*, Dr. Angela Crawford shows us how to expand our circle of compassion so we can enjoy a life well lived, while inspiring others to pursue a purpose-driven life, too. There are few things more persuasive than powerful storytelling, which is what Dr. Crawford does so beautifully, and effectively, in this ground-breaking book. To learn how to make the greatest impact on the world around you, absorb and apply the wisdom that is on full display in the pages within, to truly live your best life, while helping non-human animals live their best lives, too."—**Robert Cheeke**, *New York Times* bestselling co-author of *The Plant-Based Athlete*, and author of *The Impactful Vegan*

"How refreshing to learn I'm not the only person who has experienced a profound spiritual and emotional transformation as a result of becoming vegan! In almost 30 years living a vegan lifestyle, I've seen countless resources showing the benefits to physical health of eating a plant-based diet, but relatively few touch on the broader aspects of healing. In this wonderful, easy-to-read book, Angela Crawford, PhD, weaves the results of research she conducted with vegans from across the globe, along with her own personal and professional journey, which shows the transformative effects of living according to values of kindness and compassion to all beings. We discover how people have learned to live authentically, thrive in their personal and professional lives, and make a truly positive difference to the world. Dr. Crawford upends the myths linking veganism with sacrifice and shows how instead it's a path to transformation, abundance, and inner peace. This is a fantastic book that reveals the powerful, transformative spiritual and emotional healing that comes from embracing a vegan lifestyle. Whether you're already vegan, or simply curious, rush to get your copy now!"—**Katrina Fox**, storytelling consultant for vegan leaders, and author of *Vegan Ventures*

"A much needed and skillfully written book that I will use and share. It's a major contribution to the vegan literature, dispelling prevailing myths and revealing the truth of what veganism really is: the Swiss army knife to solving today's problems by creating a more peaceful world for all living beings, including Mother Earth.

Dr. Crawford uses her knowledge and application of psychology to guide a person who is ready for change through a transformation. Carefully weaving together her own personal story with those of others, she addresses key aspects of the behavioral change required to truly embrace a vegan lifestyle. She helps the reader align their actions with their espoused values. Behavioral change is reinforced by the benefits shown of this transformation, including ethical, health, social, existential, and consciousness-raising perspectives.

Dr. Crawford seamlessly combines facts, practical tools, and her own experience to reveal what veganism really is and the hidden benefits that only become apparent when one embraces this philosophy. She will delight the reader—whether a new vegan or one yet to be—who will discover there is no bad news about veganism, just so much to gain, which the whole world so desperately needs."—**Clare Mann**, psychologist, speaker, and author of *Vystopia: The Anguish of Being Vegan in a Non-Vegan World*

"*The Vegan Transformation* is a bold, fresh, inspired manifesto whose significance becomes more pronounced with every page. By eschewing established arguments or motivators based solely on personal health, ethics, and the environment, Dr. Angela Crawford gives veganism a broader appeal and newfound potency by illuminating its less-recognized benefits for emotional and spiritual well-being.

Crawford challenges those tired stereotypes of the restrictive or extreme lifestyle to present veganism more truthfully as an awakening that opens the world up to create deeper connections, providing a transformed sense of emotional freedom and abundance. Her extensive research and advocacy reveal the link between thinking more critically about how food gets to the plate and achieving better health and emotional fulfillment, ultimately strengthening our connection to ourselves and other beings.

Equal parts powerful and profound, erudite and accessible, at its core, *The Vegan Transformation* celebrates connection and compassion—with case studies, tools, recipes, and resources to inspire a lasting life-changing change. *The Vegan Transformation* is essential reading for a world that is out of sync with its innate humanity. It is for anyone who wants to make a deeper connection with the world around them and is curious about the transformational power of veganism. I am sending it to everyone I hold dear, daring them to expand their circle of compassion, embrace their authentic selves, and experience the benefits of alignment and transformed health."—**Todd Sinclair**, vegan influencer and author of the *Rebel Vegan Life* book series

"Angela Crawford has created a beautiful and easy-to-read guide for understanding the personal, spiritual, and emotional benefits of transitioning to a vegan lifestyle. *The Vegan Transformation* will inspire and motivate those who are newly vegan or curious about going vegan with insightful, research-backed tips and wisdom for making your vegan journey as successful as possible!"—**Sarina Farb**, vegan educator and TEDx speaker

"In *The Vegan Transformation*, Dr. Angela Crawford shares vital knowledge that invites us to explore the truth of our beliefs about health and the nature of compassion. Dr. Crawford eloquently shows us how a vegan way of life can enhance body, mind, and spirit.

Dr. Crawford's impressive original research, conducted with people from around the world, presents information that is compelling. By sharing her own powerful personal story along with the moving accounts of others, Dr. Crawford shows us how a vegan lifestyle can be successfully incorporated into one's life. This information is reinforced with practical lifestyle recommendations and references to a variety of excellent resources.

As a long-time vegan myself, I have profound appreciation for the peace that comes from knowing that no sentient being has been harmed when I enjoy a meal. I am especially grateful to Dr. Crawford for addressing this beautiful aspect of veganism. Her book is a wonderful contribution to the work of creating a healthier and more compassionate world. I am delighted to give it my highest recommendation."—**Marla Friedman**, PhD, LMHC, psychotherapist, ABAAHP, certified plant-based nutrition, author of *Love, Freedom, and Wellness: A Guide to Living an Empowered Life*

"Finally, the long-awaited book on the mental, physical, AND spiritual benefits of going vegan! Dr. Crawford brilliantly illustrates how becoming vegan IS a spiritual awakening. If the sun salutations and affirmations aren't filling that gap in your life, roll up that yoga mat and embark on a vegan journey. Create impact in ways you never imagined and gain enhanced intuition, moral alignment, and interconnectedness with all living beings. No other lifestyle trains you for adversity and saves lives. Crawford shares the challenges to expect, how to tackle them with conviction, and all the resources to sustain this lifestyle for good. The reflections and exercises inspire all readers to explore more about their own life's purpose. *The Vegan Transformation* is your definitive guide to becoming an early adopter of what will eventually be the ethical and just way to live."—**Sandra Nomoto**, hype woman for vegan leaders and author of *Vegan Marketing Success Stories*

"*The Vegan Transformation* is a must-read for vegans and non-vegans alike. Whether you are simply seeking practical ways toward vibrant health or feeling called to serve and find your most fulfilling purpose, Angela shares a message of hope and shows you how a simple compassionate change can not only transform you, but will powerfully change the world!"—**Peg Haust-Arliss**, LCSW-R, DipACT, CHHC, vegan psychotherapist, lifestyle coach, and author of *Anxiety Breakthrough: Breakout of Fear, Breakthrough to Freedom*

"Congratulations to Dr. Angela Crawford on her important book, *The Vegan Transformation*. As a long-time vegan and committed activist, I truly appreciate Angela's compassionate approach to creating change. She understands the importance of meeting people where they are and shares numerous real-life transition stories that resonate with readers, offering guidance on overcoming common struggles.

The Vegan Transformation is an excellent resource for anyone ready to embrace a healthy and humane lifestyle. It thoroughly addresses all aspects of this journey, from the benefits to the challenges faced along the way. As Dr. Crawford emphasizes, it's all about compassion—for ourselves, others, animals, and our planet. Within the vegan lifestyle lies a sense of freedom and hope for a brighter future. Angela provides a clear roadmap to help us all reach that destination."—**Cheryl Moss**, founder of Better Life for Animals and author of children's books, *Gabriel*, *Cluck*, and *Pickle*

"Dr. Angela Crawford's *The Vegan Transformation* is a gem! Crawford's writing is so engaging, and her balance of heartfelt stories with powerful insights offers clarity and connection, making it a joy to read no matter where you are on your vegan journey. More than a book about veganism, it's a profound guide to creating a life of alignment. With reflective prompts and practical applications, she invites readers to explore their values more deeply and apply what they've uncovered to bring about lasting transformation. This book is a must-read for anyone seeking a deeper sense of purpose."—**Stephanie Harter**, entrepreneur and author of *The Skinny on Eating Like You Give a Damn*

THE VEGAN TRANSFORMATION

A JOURNEY TO HEAL
YOURSELF AND THE WORLD

Angela L. Crawford, PhD

Lantern Publishing & Media • Woodstock & Brooklyn, NY

2025
Lantern Publishing & Media
PO Box 1350
Woodstock, NY 12498
www.lanternpm.org

Printed in the United States of America

Library of Congress Cataloging-in-Publication Data

Names: Crawford, Angela L., author.
Title: The vegan transformation : a journey to heal yourself and the world / Angela L. Crawford, PhD.
Description: Woodstock, NY ; Brooklyn, NY : Lantern Publishing & Media, 2025. | Includes bibliographical references.
Identifiers: LCCN 2024034693 (print) | LCCN 2024034694 (ebook) | ISBN 9781590567432 (paperback) | ISBN 9781590567449 (epub)
Subjects: LCSH: Veganism—Philosophy. | Nutrition. | Diet—Moral and ethical aspects.
Classification: LCC TX392 .C778 2025 (print) | LCC TX392 (ebook) | DDC 613.2/622—dc23/eng/20240910
LC record available at https://lccn.loc.gov/2024034693
LC ebook record available at https://lccn.loc.gov/2024034694

DISCLAIMER

This book is designed to provide accurate information and resources regarding the subject matter covered. Any content or opinions given should not substitute for medical advice and services from a trained healthcare professional. Please consult with a qualified medical provider regarding healthcare decisions and treatment. If you take medications for a health condition, it is important that you discuss any dietary changes with your physician, as changes in your diet may impact the amount of medication needed. In addition, it is essential to seek consultation from your medical provider for any medication changes (i.e., starting, stopping, or altering dosages). Neither the publisher nor the writer may be held liable for the use of any information contained in this book.

To all who dare to expand their circle of compassion.

CONTENTS

FOREWORD

Victoria Moran

Going vegan is like falling in love: you can't know how it feels until it happens to you. Of course, every romantic novice looks toward finding *the one* with rapt anticipation. Few omnivores, however, daydream about how fabulous life will be once they get past meat, fish, eggs, and dairy products. And yet, as Dr. Angela Crawford and the many vegans she interviewed for this book attest, adoption of a plant-based diet and cruelty-free lifestyle almost invariably elevates the experience of living on Earth.

This means that we're not talking merely about a vegan shift, a vegan conversion, or even a vegan commitment, laudable as these are. We're talking about *the vegan transformation*, a unique and as yet minimally examined phenomenon that endows those who encounter it with a renewed sense of purpose, heightened self-esteem, and often an inexplicable belief that things can get better, even when the means for bringing this about are not immediately forthcoming.

This is extraordinary because embarking on the vegan path happens after one becomes aware of the tremendous suffering of innocent land and sea creatures for human food, clothing, research, sport, and amusement. While this certainly causes deep sadness for those who care enough to change their lives to help stop it, relatively few give in to despair. Instead, vegans by and large transmute hopelessness into action. They seem motivated by a boundless fount of energy. It could be the kale, but I think it's the transformation.

This sort of reinvention isn't something you can learn or something you can buy, any more than a caterpillar needs to seek out a YouTube video on how to become a butterfly. Transformation happens for vegans because this life choice invites it.

We generally reserve the term *transformation* for a complete change of attitude and demeanor, rather like that of Ebeneezer Scrooge after a sobering look at Christmas past, present, and future. The vegan transformation, compellingly detailed in this book, comes about after a look at the following:

- Elements of our past, at the food and lifestyle choices we absorbed, usually without question, from family and culture
- Assessment of the present, that having scrambled eggs for breakfast, a cheeseburger for lunch, and grilled chicken for dinner looks "normal," but does, in fact, cause suffering and violent, premature death for innocent animals. It also plays a role in world hunger, exacerbates climate change, and is no friend of our arteries.
- Embracing a future vision of personal health and a peaceful planet where the rights of all livingkind are honored and respected.

Like Dickens' fictional character, we go from "Bah humbug!" to "God bless us everyone" in the real world.

This doesn't mean that veganism is the key to endless bliss or even perfect health, although ample science attests that eating whole plant foods is the nutritional gold standard. What it does, in my understanding—an understanding now deepened by the information in this book—is trigger a psychic reset. It's a way to start over. As Franz Kafka famously said to fish in an aquarium, "I can finally look at you in peace. I do not eat you anymore." And, yes, today's dedicated animal rights proponents wouldn't be visiting an aquarium, one more place where animals are held against their will. But compassion is not a changeless, rule-bound catechism. It is, rather, a living and growing concept that evolves throughout our lives and in human history.

In my life, the vegan metamorphosis led to an incredible lightness that I believe was the lifting of guilt I hadn't realized I was carrying. It also brought an overwhelming desire to mitigate suffering and create peace. I made the switch in my dietary and lifestyle choices because it felt like the right thing to do, but I didn't expect such a positive realignment of my relationship with myself and the world around me. I didn't expect to fall in love. And yet I was recast into a person with a calling—that's not confined to prospective clergy, I've learned—and I fell head over heels in love with the essence of life shared by all beings. This happened for me over forty years ago. No one ever explained it until now: *The Vegan Transformation*.

So, my friend, I trust you will delight in this long-awaited book by an author who is the "real deal." She walks her talk, and as you read these pages, you'll hear her wise and patient counsel. A grand adventure awaits. You've picked up the right book, at the right time.

—**Victoria Moran**, author of *Main Street Vegan* and *Age Like a Yogi*; director, Main Street Vegan Academy; host, Main Street Vegan Podcast

INTRODUCTION

What is vegan transformation?

If you are picking up this book, perhaps you hope to create a transformation in your life. Maybe you are curious about adopting a plant-based or vegan lifestyle. You may wonder, as the book title suggests: *Can becoming vegan really usher in transformation and healing?* Many of us have areas of our personal lives that we wish to, perhaps magically, transform for the better. And when we witness distressing global tragedies, natural disasters, polarization and division, and large-scale suffering around us, we also long for transformative healing in our world.

> *Transformation*: A thorough or dramatic change in character, condition, or form. Closely aligned with the word *metamorphosis*, which is "An abrupt and startling change induced by, or as if by, magic or a supernatural power," much like how a caterpillar transforms into a butterfly.[1]

I want to share a message of hope—that a simple, compassionate change in what you eat can hold the secret for greater health and emotional fulfillment, while also protecting animals, humans, and the planet. I invite you to read on, to discover the healing power of vegan living for mind, body, and spirit, as shared through my story and the stories of other vegans, all grounded in a vast body of research on plant-powered living and wellness.

What are you seeking?

Before we get started, take a moment to think about the healing or transformations that would make a positive difference in your life. Consider the following possibilities:

- Healing from a medical condition and reclaiming active, vibrant health
- Reaching your healthiest, ideal weight and feeling more energetic, youthful, and physically fit
- Living a life that is deeply authentic and expresses your truest self
- Overcoming obstacles to follow your dreams
- Finding and serving your highest, most fulfilling purpose
- Creating and nurturing meaningful relationships
- Life-changing spiritual awakening or growth

As you read this book, you will be invited to consider the healing that you long for, both in your personal life and for our world. You will be guided to explore the ways that a plant-powered lifestyle, along with inner growth and other healthy changes, can support you on your healing journey. Together, we will head off to discover—through learning, inner exploration, and practice—what helps *you* to flourish in mind, body, and spirit.

There are many ways that we can transform our lives, some with more meaningful results than others. What I love about *vegan transformation* is that it empowers fulfilling inner changes, and also your living more compassionately and lightly on our planet. You'll come to realize that caring for yourself and caring for others are complementary actions that affirm your personal well-being *and* the health of our planet. This has been one of the most surprising, fulfilling, and inspiring discoveries of my own vegan transformation.

My vegan transformation

First, a little background about me. I have long been fascinated by the mysteries of life and nature. From a young age, I was a voracious reader, with a love for mystery novels and historical fiction, as well as non-fiction books about personal growth, self-esteem, healing, and spirituality. These interests led me on a path, first as a journalism major, later transitioning to psychology and completing a Ph.D. in clinical psychology. All through my life, I have worked on my own personal healing in areas such as healthy lifestyle habits, self-esteem, spiritual growth, finances, emotional well-being, and relationships. Through my past work as a psychotherapist for twenty-five years, I helped hundreds of individuals on their healing journeys, addressing stress, trauma, and emotional issues, while creating more meaningful and fulfilling lives.

One of the most transformative experiences in my own life was becoming vegan. It started when I became vegetarian in late 2006, after learning about the working conditions in meat processing plants from a PBS special. I was appalled at the treatment of workers, who suffered terrible working conditions and frequent injuries. Many were immigrants who struggled financially and had few options for other employment. Learning about this led me to think more critically about how my food got to me. And then I thought, "If I don't like how the workers are treated, what about the animals?" I soon began buying plant-based cookbooks and reading every book in my local library about vegetarianism and veganism.

Becoming a plant-based eater was a big transition for me. Although I had always loved animals and nature, I had never considered the process by which my food came to me. I never thought about the impact of animal agriculture or realized the suffering that animals experienced in factory farms. I didn't know the devastating effects of the animal agriculture industry on the environment and our planet. Growing up in Iowa farm country, I only saw the cows grazing in the fields. I didn't know about the large-scale factory farms that raised, bred, and slaughtered billions of animals, since these were kept well out of sight.

I also struggled with my eating patterns for many of my earlier years. I was not a healthy eater. From a very young age, I ate a lot of comfort foods: chocolates, sweets, and salty snacks. When I moved out on my own, my main meals were microwave dinners and other convenience foods. Once I finally started to cook, I stuck to a limited repertoire of go-to meals, always including some type of meat (usually chicken) and perhaps a small serving of veggies in a buttery sauce. Like many people, I believed I needed to eat meat and dairy to thrive. This is what I had been taught by my school, my doctors, and what was presented in the media. But after watching that PBS special, I began to question what I had been taught. As I began researching the ins and outs of vegetarian living, I learned not only that I could thrive physically with a plant-based diet, but also that this way of living was much kinder to animals and the planet. This ultimately led to my adopting a vegan lifestyle, free of all animal products.

My path to veganism transformed me from an unhealthy eater to a proficient cook, creating delicious and nutritious plant-based meals and enjoying improved health and energy. I found that I actually enjoyed, and became passionate about, cooking. I went from being someone who barely cooked for myself (sometimes eating only cheese and crackers for dinner) to making weekly vegetarian soups and other plant-based dishes to share with my partner and his family.

I also found my voice. As someone who identifies as an introvert, I lived a private and quiet life. My work as a psychotherapist certainly allowed for that, as I worked in a private practice, doing individual and small group psychotherapy. My daily routine centered around deeply meaningful, emotionally impactful therapeutic work with clients. I didn't have a website or social media, and I didn't enjoy public speaking. I kept a low public profile.

Becoming vegan changed all of that. Within six months of my committing to a fully vegan lifestyle, I attended Main Street Vegan Academy (MSVA) in New York City and became a Certified Vegan Lifestyle Coach and Educator. There I met the inspiring founder of MSVA, Victoria Moran, and other passionate vegan teachers and attendees. Through the course of this life-changing class, I learned to share my story with greater confidence. I also learned more about all the reasons that being vegan aligns so well with my values. The more I learned, the more I became committed to sharing this transformative way of living with others. Although I am still an introvert, my passion for veganism overshadowed my natural reserve.

Within a year I had started a website and blog focused on psychology and veganism, writing on topics such as navigating social challenges as a vegan, thriving emotionally, and the benefits of veganism for mind, body, and spirit. I found myself engaged in public speaking when I was invited to do presentations and interviews about these issues, something I couldn't have imagined previously. I took a plant-based nutrition course and later taught an online vegan cooking course. I met vegans from all over the world through various online networking groups and social media. In honoring my core values and daring to speak out about these values with others, I found a like-hearted tribe, along with greater confidence, peace, and fulfillment.

Why I wrote this book

As I conversed with vegans around the globe, I became fascinated by how they reported their own transformations since embarking on a vegan lifestyle. Some reported dramatic physical healing, while others reported greater peace and well-being, spiritual growth, and/or a compelling sense of purpose and contribution.

These vegan transformations intrigued me, and this led to my book research. Non-vegans often see veganism as extreme, restrictive, or depriving. I can relate. Before I shifted to a plant-based lifestyle, I wondered, "What would a vegetarian or vegan eat?" I thought it was about giving things up. And yet, once I became vegan, what I experienced was a sense of abundance, freedom, and fulfillment. Many other vegans express these same feelings. I wanted to study and capture this paradox—perhaps it might inspire those who are curious about veganism to embrace this life-affirming path.

My background as a psychologist made me curious about the process of change and what leads people to consider a vegan lifestyle. How can we inspire others, especially when this lifestyle can be lifesaving? In the United States, we are facing an unprecedented health crisis, with an increasing prevalence of lifestyle-related disease and escalating costs of medical care. Healthcare costs in the United States are almost twose that of other industrialized nations,[2] while our life expectancy (a key indicator of healthcare outcomes) has actually declined in recent years.[3] How do we support others to become aware of, and open to, the very information that could help them—and our communities—be healthier?

I was also curious from the standpoint of compassion. In my work as a therapist, I had learned that those who were abusive to children quite often showed cruelty toward animals as well. How we treat non-human animals and how we treat other humans is inextricably interconnected. Our ability to experience compassion for animals has been recognized as a positive indicator of mental health, while deliberate cruelty to animals is often associated with antisocial behaviors and can be a predictor of violence toward others.

The process of killing animals for food is incredibly violent, but we, as consumers, are shielded from this violence. The convenience and visual appeal of our food marketing and delivery systems have insulated and conditioned us to turn away from acknowledging this brutality, even those of us who are compassionate and care about animals. However, wise figures throughout history, going back as far as Pythagoras in 570 BCE, have advocated a vegetarian diet for creating a more humane and peaceful world.

After awakening to the many benefits of a vegan lifestyle, I wondered what took me so long to embrace something that was clearly aligned with my values of compassion and kindness toward others. In addition, I was disheartened to find that often I was the sole vegan in my professional networks, even among very compassionate and caring colleagues in fields such as psychology, medicine, education, holistic health, spiritual counseling, and coaching.

At the present time, only about 3 percent of the global population identifies as vegan.[4] I wondered, how can this gap exist when there is so much research showing the health benefits of a plant-based lifestyle and demonstrating that animal agriculture is the leading contributor to climate change and environmental degradation? How could so many of us who are educated, conscious, and compassionate not connect with the incredible suffering that animals go through in the food system? And in other systems as well, such as research and entertainment? Why are we so blind to this?

Through my research, I hoped to learn more about the psychological and spiritual impacts of a vegan lifestyle. I had witnessed incredible healing and transformation in many vegans I knew. Was this common for other vegans? I hoped that this research might empower and support those who were curious about being plant-based but have concerns: "Is this lifestyle doable? Enjoyable? Fulfilling?" There are many books on the healing power of a plant-based lifestyle for physical health, but there are fewer about the psychological, emotional, and mental health benefits. I researched and wrote this book to help fill in this gap.

Who is this book for?

If you identify with any of the following, this book is written for you!

- You're curious about a vegan or plant-based lifestyle—whether for personal health and wellness, compassion, ethics, the environment, or all of the above—but you're not sure how to thrive with a vegan lifestyle. As you read on, you will discover inspiration and tools for how to become plant-based in a way that is doable and feels good on all levels—mind, body, and spirit.
- You're afraid that going plant-based or vegan would be too difficult and restrictive, that it means depriving yourself or giving things up. The research and inspiring vegan stories will show you the abundance that is possible and how you can experience it too.
- You're compassionate and care about making the world a better place and want to include your own well-being in this venture. From the principles and tools offered, you can discover how to contribute meaningfully in ways that are fueled by self-kindness and self-care.
- You want to take charge of your own well-being, through healthy plant-based living and positive lifestyle practices. Each chapter teaches principles and actions for greater empowerment and holistic wellness.
- You're already plant-based or vegan, and looking for inspiration, support, guidance, and skills to be a more empowered, joyful, and impactful vegan. Thank you for all you are already doing to contribute to a healthier and more compassionate world. May this book empower you on your continued path!

My research with vegans

I began research for this book in spring 2021, creating an online survey to explore the impacts of a vegan lifestyle on emotional, social, and spiritual well-being. I surveyed about 350 vegans and followed up with 75 in-depth interviews to learn how they have benefited emotionally and spiritually from a vegan lifestyle. I also explored the emotional challenges that come with being vegan, and how participants coped with them. Those participating in the survey included residents of the United States, United Kingdom, Canada, Australia, the Netherlands, France, India, Israel, and Japan.

I coded the data from the survey responses to identify the most common themes and experiences reported by participants. The core themes that emerged are ones that many would agree are foundational to a life well lived. They are relevant to vegans as well as to non-vegans— and are qualities that psychology and related fields view as important for human flourishing. The most common benefits that my research respondents reported were: as follows

- The peace of living in alignment with core values
- Greater compassion and empathy
- Increased sense of meaning and purpose
- Personal fulfillment
- Meaningful connections with others who share the same values
- Empowerment over health
- A deeper experience of being connected to nature and all life

In this book, I devote a chapter to each of these themes, drawing on the specific experiences and stories of my research participants, as well as the broader research literature, to illustrate the relevance and impact of each theme. I will share more about this shortly.

There are some caveats to this research that need to be mentioned. This was an exploratory study to learn more from vegans about their emotional and spiritual experiences. This is a descriptive and qualitative study; thus, no causal relationships can be determined. (This means, the data can't determine what *caused* any changes reported by study participants). Participants were recruited through invitations on

LinkedIn and Facebook and various vegan online groups. This was a relatively small sample, and it was not randomly selected; therefore, it is not representative of all vegans. Vegans are a diverse group of people, and not all vegans experience the feelings and perspectives shared here through my research.

However, the responses in my surveys captured an experience that is common for many vegans, an experience that provides a path of possibility. *This is the possibility of creating a meaningful, healthy, and fulfilling life—a life that also contributes to a kinder, healthier world.* While there are no guarantees that becoming vegan will bring these qualities into your life, perhaps you may find, as many of my survey participants did, that deciding to leave animals off the dinner plate is one of the most healing and life-changing choices you can make.

What this book covers

Starting your journey

We start out in Chapter One by looking at the ethical, environmental, and medical implications of our food choices, how veganism provides a solution in many of these areas, and why these issues are increasingly urgent. I also address some misconceptions about veganism, clarify definitions, and introduce the transformative possibilities that you can experience through plant-powered, vegan living.

The path of vegan transformation

Chapters Two through Eight discuss the seven key transformative themes that emerged through my research with vegans, and how you can cultivate these qualities in your own life:

- Chapter Two: The Courage to Live Your Values
- Chapter Three: Expand Your Circle of Compassion
- Chapter Four: Connect with Deeper Meaning and Purpose
- Chapter Five: Create Authentic Fulfillment
- Chapter Six: The Power of True Connection
- Chapter Seven: Take Charge of Your Health
- Chapter Eight: Discover Your Interconnectedness with Life

Each chapter provides background information and research about the theme being covered, as well as survey responses and stories from my interviewees that illustrate how these themes touched their lives. Through their stories, you will discover inspiring examples of how plant-powered living can empower wellness in mind, body, and spirit. At the end of each chapter, I offer action steps and reflection exercises for you to engage with so that you can experience these healing benefits in your own life. These exercises aim to connect you with your own core values and your own inner wisdom so that you can move forward in ways that are best for you.

From Awakening to Action

In Chapter Nine, I share behavior-change principles to empower you to transition to a vegan lifestyle and/or make other healthy lifestyle changes. Chapter Ten identifies some of the emotional and social challenges vegans may face and how to navigate these successfully. Last of all, in Chapter Eleven, I explore how your own healing journey can contribute to larger healing in our world.

Resources and Recipes

In the back of the book, I provide all kinds of resources for wherever you are on your plant-powered journey, including suggestions for books, websites, and documentaries that cover various aspects of plant-based and vegan living. In addition, you will find a small recipe section. When I told my non-vegan friends about writing this book, they all asked, "Will there be recipes?" In response, I invited some of my research participants who have cookbooks, vegan food businesses, and/or recipe blogs to share a few of their awesome recipes. Please check them out!

What this book does not cover

Just as described, this book focuses on the mind-body-spirit healing and wellness that can be experienced alongside a vegan lifestyle, and core principles and practices that help create this. It is designed to inspire you, and to help you follow your most aligned path. It does *not* teach the specifics of plant-based nutrition or detailed how-to skills of becoming vegan, such as setting up a vegan kitchen, vegan cooking, or finding vegan products. These are beyond the scope of this book. However, I offer numerous suggestions in the Resources section to find more information about these areas. As you read and explore the ideas in this book, you may find that uncovering your inspiration for change (your WHY) seamlessly guides you toward the HOW of transitioning that works best for you.

Let's get started

Creating this book has been quite a long journey—and a path of discovery for me. After speaking with many inspiring individuals through my research surveys and interviews, I am both intrigued and uplifted by their experiences of growth, healing, and transformation. Now, I am super excited to share these discoveries with you! Let's dive in and explore the possibilities for healing yourself and the world through a plant-powered, vegan lifestyle.

PART ONE

STARTING YOUR JOURNEY

CHAPTER 1

THE TRANSFORMATIVE POWER OF A VEGAN LIFESTYLE

> "By choosing to eat life-giving rather than life-taking foods, we're saying yes to our values of wellness and health, of peace and nonviolence, of kindness and compassion."
> —**Colleen Patrick-Goudreau** in *The Joyful Vegan*[1]

> "I believe the path to veganism is like a homecoming—to return to your original compassionate self."
> —**Todd Sinclair** in *Rebel Vegan Life*[2]

Have you ever felt pulled to make some kind of life change, maybe even a change that surprised you? Maybe it was an inner knowing that it was time to leave your job, start down a new career path, end a relationship, or finally take charge of your health. You may have felt an inner call, a sense that you needed to take action, even though you weren't sure exactly how it would all work out. Or perhaps circumstances lined up so that you saw no other choice but to launch onto a new path, unknown and uncertain. This call from the deepest parts of us often gives us the opportunity to become a truer version of ourselves. It can lead us down pathways that initially we are somewhat hesitant to take, but ultimately seem very right, even exhilarating.

This has happened many times in my life. One example is when I changed majors from journalism to psychology midway through my junior year of college. I had always envisioned myself as a writer. I have loved reading and writing since childhood, and the main vision I had for my future was to be an author who wrote books and feature articles for a magazine. However, a confluence of events revealed that something deep inside of me had a different idea about my future. I found myself fascinated by my psychology courses, the workings of the human mind, and the possibility of helping others. A chance meeting with a friend led me to enroll in the Psychology Honors Program at my university. In addition to being drawn to the subject matter, I found that this path was more aligned with my reserved nature, rather than having to constantly seek out a story to write. This was a field of study that I was passionate about, that would naturally lead me to meaningful conversations and collaborations with colleagues and clients. It would also immerse me in the subject area I was most drawn to write about. And of course, as it turns out, life has a way of going full circle. Here I am, finally writing that book I have always dreamed about.

Becoming vegan was one of those surprising life changes as well. My Midwestern upbringing taught me that meat and dairy were absolute necessities, that I couldn't survive (and certainly couldn't thrive) without them. I had meat for most of my meals; I thought something was missing if it wasn't there. I thought I needed it for energy, to have enough protein, and to balance out my sugar highs. On top of that, life felt too overwhelming to take on any major dietary changes, anything that would require extra energy beyond eating what was tasty, familiar, and convenient. I had met only a few vegans, and I couldn't imagine what they ate or how it could possibly sustain them. I couldn't see being vegetarian or vegan as a possibility in my own life.

My path to becoming vegan was one of awakening, bit by bit. In retrospect, I see that first I was shown how it could be possible. After eating delicious, satisfying, beautifully presented vegetarian meals at a conference center that served primarily plant-based cuisine, I said to myself, "I think I could eat this way, if I had a chef to cook for me." I still couldn't see myself taking on cooking, but I now knew I wouldn't starve or die if I ate this way. A few months later, my stepdaughter was home for Thanksgiving break, during her first semester of college. She recently had gone vegetarian, and at Thanksgiving dinner, she ate all the vegetable dishes and mashed potatoes, but no turkey. She seemed to enjoy the meal as much as any of us. Again, I felt a new glimmer of possibility. It was less than a month later that I saw a show on PBS about slaughterhouse workers that made me really think about the food I ate and the whole process of how it arrived on the supermarket shelf. This led me to buy my first plant-based cookbook and follow an unexpected path of change.

What I subsequently discovered—about food, the systems that produce it, and the vast ripple effects of our eating choices—was so compelling that I literally couldn't stop reading and learning. This led me to become vegetarian, and several years later, vegan. I discovered that becoming vegan is not just a dietary choice, like the latest low-carb diet craze or cutting calories to lose weight. It does involve changing what you eat, but it is so much more. It's one of those rare life opportunities, where in changing something as basic as what you eat, you have the potential not only to optimize your own physical, emotional, and spiritual wellness, but also to contribute to healing many of the larger problems that face our world today.

Why vegan?

As we watch the news or scan social media, it seems that the problems that face us globally are ever-growing: climate change, natural disasters, pandemics, wars, hunger and food insecurity, disease, environmental destruction, and acts of violence. Many of us feel overwhelmed and a deep sense of sorrow as we witness the devastating effects of these events. And it may seem that we have very little power over the catastrophes and crises that our world faces. Many of these issues are of such magnitude and complexity that our individual actions don't appear to have much impact.

However, one thing that many of us—at least, those of us with adequate financial resources—do have control over is the choice of what we eat and what we purchase. These are choices we make daily that have a huge (although often unseen) impact. A plant-based diet and lifestyle provides the missing puzzle piece for addressing many of the troubling issues in our world: healing chronic disease, environmental and climate healing, preventing pandemics, and cultivating a more compassionate and less violent society. You may be wondering, how can something so seemingly basic as our food choices have such an impact on these global challenges? And why plant-based? How does this make a difference?

While moving to a plant-based diet may not heal *all* the issues we are facing, it has the potential to address many problems that threaten our personal and global well-being. I will review some of them next.

Healing and reversing disease

Let's start with our physical health. The rates of chronic disease, particularly cardiovascular disease, are rising to epidemic levels in the United States. Many of you likely have loved ones who are suffering from some type of chronic medical condition, or perhaps you are struggling with your own health issues. Moving to a solely plant-based diet can be one of the best choices you can make for your overall health and well-being. A strong body of empirical evidence finds that a plant-strong diet focused on whole foods can treat or manage many of the chronic diseases we face today, such as coronary heart disease, Type 2 diabetes, and autoimmune disease. Plant-based diets have been shown to not only prevent, but reverse many of these diseases. These studies find that eating an abundance of whole plant foods (such as fruits, veggies, greens, beans, lentils, whole grains, nuts, and seeds) while eliminating meat, dairy, and highly processed foods, decreases your risk of many health issues that are prevalent today.[3]

Plant foods are anti-inflammatory and rich in nutrients and antioxidants, provide ample fiber, have less saturated fat, and contain no cholesterol. A high-nutrient, whole-food vegan diet appears to help reverse early stages of cognitive decline and reduces the risk for developing Alzheimer's disease.[4] On top of that, many athletes have discovered that a plant-powered diet can improve athletic performance and fitness.[5] Some wonderful books for learning more about regaining and revitalizing health through a plant-based diet include *The China Study*, *How Not to Die*, *Eat for Life*, and *Fiber-Fueled*.[6] Or check out the documentaries *Forks over Knives*, *What the Health*, or *The Game Changers*.[7]

Compassion for animals

Being vegan is also a stance of kindness and compassion for animals. Many of us care deeply about our companion animals, such as dogs, cats, and horses. However, we are raised from a young age to turn a blind eye to the farm animals who are raised for food. We forget (or are never taught) that these animals are sentient beings who have intelligence, personalities, feelings, and complex social relationships. Like other sentient beings, they seek comfort and try to avoid pain. It's heart-breaking to realize that over ninety billion land animals are slaughtered worldwide each year for food. If you include sea creatures, these numbers are in the trillions. Ten billion land animals are slaughtered each year in the United States alone. And most of this meat, over 98 percent, comes from industrialized agriculture, also known as factory farming.[8]

Animals raised on factory farms live in extremely confined, crowded, miserable, unsanitary conditions for the short duration of their lives. Most are given no access to sunlight or the outdoors. They are forced to endure painful procedures without anesthesia. Their short lives end in an inhumane and violent slaughter process. Sometimes it's hard to grasp how horrific these conditions are until you see pictures or video footage from the inside of factory farms and slaughterhouses. Because "Ag-Gag" laws have made it a criminal offense to take photos or videos inside these facilities, we would have no knowledge of what goes on inside if not for the courage and commitment of undercover activists and journalists. One might wonder why these Ag-Gag laws were designed, other than to hide the ugly truth from the public.[9]

Some of you may be thinking, "I try to eat humane meat, so it's kinder to animals." First, just to be clear—most meat comes from industrialized factory farming. However, even farms that do describe themselves as humane may not be as kind to animals as you think. When you look more closely, many "humane" farms still engage in cruel and painful practices in the process of raising and breeding animals, and very often the animals end up in the same slaughterhouses as factory-farmed animals.[10] In addition, when you consider the amount of meat that's currently consumed worldwide, "humane farming" is not a sustainable or viable option to meet current demands, in terms of land, water, and resource use.

Beyond animal agriculture, there are other industries that routinely exploit and harm animals. This includes testing and research that is conducted on animals; entertainment such as rodeos and circuses; mass breeding in puppy mills; and the leather, wool, and down industries. As we gain greater awareness, we can use the power of our purchases to choose not to support industries that harm animals, and instead make cruelty-free buying choices whenever possible. To learn more about how your food and other buying choices affect animals, you may wish to visit the websites of the Humane Society of the United States (HSUS) and People for the Ethical Treatment of Animals (PETA), or read books that share about the realities of factory farming, such as *Diet for a New America* or *Eating Animals*.[11]

Caring for the environment

In recent years, we have faced unprecedented weather events, including catastrophic flooding, devastating wildfires, and hurricanes and tornadoes that cause vast destruction. We are also experiencing rising sea levels, record heat, droughts, water shortages, pollution, ocean dead zones, species extinction, and soil erosion. It's hard to ignore the growing impacts of climate change and environmental degradation. Increasingly, they are affecting our daily lives.

These environmental problems are not inevitable. What is often not mentioned, even by climate and environmental activists, is the huge role that intensive animal agriculture plays in climate change and the destruction of the environment. Livestock production is responsible for more of the world's greenhouse gas emissions than the entire transport industry, including cars, planes, transport trucks, and boats. A 2009 report by the Worldwatch Institute estimated that at least 51 percent of greenhouse gasses can be attributed to animal agriculture.[12] Other sources estimate that this percentage may actually be much higher when all contributing factors are considered.[13] Eating a plant-based diet, while eliminating meat, fish, and dairy, can cut your carbon footprint in half.[14]

Animal agriculture is also a huge contributor to deforestation, which further accelerates climate change. Our forests, particularly the vast Amazon rainforests, counterbalance and absorb the carbon dioxide that is emitted through greenhouse gasses, lessening their impact. The rainforests also help to moderate weather and precipitation cycles. More than 80 percent of the cutting or burning of forests is done to support livestock production, mostly for grazing and growing animal feed. The land cleared for meat-based diets is a major contributor to global biodiversity loss and species extinction as well.[15]

It takes enormous resources (land, food, and water) to raise and feed billions of animals each year. About half of the planet's land surface is devoted to animal agriculture (e.g., grazing; growing soy, corn, and grains for farmed animals; and animal confinement structures). Over forty percent of the world's grain is fed to livestock, while one billion people go to bed hungry every night. We grow more than enough food to feed our global population, yet many people don't have access to adequate nutrition.[16] Since the book *Diet for a Small Planet* was first published in 1971, there has been increasing awareness of the inefficiency of animal-sourced foods when it comes to feeding the human population. While the exact ratio differs depending on the size of the animal, on average, for every 100 calories of crops fed to livestock, we get back only about 30 calories of animal protein.[17] In many cases, with larger animals, there is even less efficiency. Frances Moore Lappe, author of *Diet for a Small Planet*, found that it takes about sixteen pounds of feed to produce one pound of beef.[18]

Livestock production uses immense amounts of water, accounting for about 70 percent of all water use.[19] Many people now live in areas that face increasing water scarcity. We try to conserve water in various ways, such as doing fewer loads of laundry or taking shorter showers. However, when it comes to water use, shorter showers can't offset the enormous amounts of water required for raising farmed animals. For example, it takes about *1800 gallons of water* to produce *one pound of beef*. That is equivalent to forty loads of laundry or twenty-six showers.[20]

In addition, animal agriculture is a major contributor to water and air pollution. Large-scale animal agriculture produces far more waste than can be used for fertilizer. Animal waste from factory farming often ends up being stored in lagoons and/or sprayed into the air (creating health hazards for workers and those who are unfortunate enough to live nearby), and leaches into lakes, rivers, and other water sources, poisoning our water and creating ocean dead zones.[21]

Many people view eating fish as a solution to these environmental problems. However, our oceans are being overfished at a rate that many experts say far exceeds the ability for species to replenish. In addition, large-scale industrialized fishing uses large trawlers that scrape up everything in their path, killing many creatures that were not intended to be caught in the nets, such as dolphins and seals, and destroying coral reefs and other sea habitats. Fish farming has its own problems, with extreme overcrowding of fish, rapid spread of disease, and parasite infestations, all of which require added chemicals and antibiotics to help combat them.[22]

It doesn't have to be this way! We can help to heal our environment by changing what we eat. According to the authors of the book, *Eat for the Planet*, one person eating plant-based (i.e., no meat, fish, eggs, or dairy) saves 1,500 gallons of water, forty-five pounds of grain, and thirty square feet of forest *each day*. Only one-sixth of an acre is needed to feed a vegan for a full year—while a meat-eater requires eighteen times that much land.[23] When it comes to living more sustainably and with less of an impact on our planet, going plant-based is a no-brainer. To learn more about the impact of your food choices on the environment, you may wish to check out the documentaries *Cowspiracy*, *Seaspiracy*, and *Eating Our Way to Extinction*,[24] or read books such as *Eat for the Planet* and *Food Is Climate*.[25]

Preventing pandemics

Eating a plant-exclusive diet also helps to prevent pandemics. The recent COVID-19 pandemic has affected countless lives, causing untimely deaths, long-term health effects, increased mental health issues, and lingering economic consequences. At the time of writing this book, COVID-19 has caused nearly seven million deaths since its onset in early 2020.[26] This virus is still with us, mutating into new COVID variants. Scientists warn that an even more lethal and transmissible virus is likely to impact us at some point in the not-too-distant future.

When we examine the root cause of infectious diseases, we find that most are zoonotic, meaning that they originate from animals and are passed onto humans. This includes diseases that are newer to us, as well as those that have been around for a long time: influenza (a.k.a. the flu), HIV and AIDS, bird flu, swine flu, measles, and even the common cold. The way that we produce food has increased our exposure to these zoonotic viruses. Due to continued encroachment on natural ecosystems, along with the implementation of intensive animal agriculture practices, we are increasingly at risk for interspecies disease transmission. It is not just wet markets or live markets that create this risk. The crowded, unsanitary conditions for factory farmed animals make them highly vulnerable to becoming infected and spreading these pathogens.[27] This is highlighted by recent increases in avian flu among chickens and turkeys being raised for food.

Our food choices not only play a key role in the likelihood of future pandemics; they also impact our individual susceptibility to severe illness when we are exposed to infectious disease. A report published in the *British Journal of Medicine* examined dietary patterns and COVID-19 severity among 2,884 front-line healthcare workers. The researchers found, after controlling for possible confounding variables, that those who consumed a plant-based diet had a *73 percent lower risk* of experiencing moderate to severe COVID-19, compared to meat-eaters. While the rates of contracting COVID-19 did not differ significantly among dietary groups in this study, those who ate plant-based were strongly protected against more severe forms of the disease.[28] In addition, a recent study of 702 Brazilians found that those who consumed a vegetarian, vegan, or predominantly plant-based diet had 39 percent lower odds of *contracting* COVID-19, compared to those who consumed an omnivorous diet.[29] A strong body of research finds that a plant-centered diet boosts our immunity to help fight infections and other diseases.[30]

To learn more about decreasing the risk of future pandemics through plant-powered living, I encourage you to check out Dr. Michael Greger's book, *How to Survive a Pandemic*,[31] as well as his NutritionFacts.org website, which reviews and summarizes peer-reviewed research on nutrition and health.[32]

Ethical, moral, and spiritual values

And last of all, eating plant-based is aligned with many of our ethical and spiritual values. Most spiritual and religious traditions teach the importance of nonviolence or *ahimsa*. Ahimsa is an ancient Indian principle of holding respect for all living beings and avoiding harm or violence whenever it is in our power to do so.[33] Most major religions agree on a core message of treating others as we would want to be treated, showing kindness, and not harming or killing others, particularly the vulnerable. Choosing not to consume animals or their products is an active stance toward compassion, nonviolence, and the ethical treatment of sentient beings.

When we consider the ethics of our food choices, it's important to note that these choices affect the well-being of humans as well as animals. Our industrialized animal agriculture system disproportionately causes harm to more vulnerable human populations. For example, workers in factory farms and slaughterhouses generally earn low wages, while being subjected to incredibly hazardous, unsafe, and unsanitary conditions. Many are poor, marginalized, and/or immigrants, and have little power to advocate for better pay or safer work conditions. In addition, the air and water pollution resulting from factory farms is more likely to affect impoverished communities that don't have the social or political clout to fight back. On top of this, factory farming uses vast resources, amplifying food and water shortages for poor and vulnerable populations.[34] Thus, moving toward a more compassionate, just, and environmentally sustainable food system has moral and ethical impacts for both human and non-human animals.

Why now?

To sum up, our food choices have enormous consequences when it comes to health, ethics, and the environment. We can take our power back by choosing a plant-powered, vegan lifestyle to help create a healthier life and a healthier world. This choice is especially important now, as we are reaching a tipping point with many of these problems. Our climate and environmental issues are worsening, leading many experts to predict that the damage could become irreversible in a very short time, leading to devastating consequences. In recent years, we have witnessed increasing weather-related disasters, including historic drought, tragic wildfires, rising sea levels, and record flooding. At the same time, we are faced with escalating rates of degenerative diseases, accompanied by the ever-rising cost of healthcare. And amidst all of this, we are plagued with increasing mental health and substance abuse problems, growing social disconnection, and socioeconomic and racial inequity.

Underlying many of these crises is the proverbial elephant (or cow) in the room[35] that we are blind to or don't want to see—that is, the vast numbers of animals killed each year, reaching previously unimaginable levels due to industrialization that turns farms into factories. Because we are raised to believe that eating animals is something we *need* to do, we continue to eat foods that harm animals, our health, our emotional well-being, and our planet. Most of us never critically examine or question the system that produces our food, a system that is often at odds with values that most of us hold dear, such as compassion, kindness, health, wellness, sustainability, and justice. Through our choice to eat meat, we are in effect paying others to do violent, cruel, and often dangerous work in slaughterhouses and factory farms that most of us would never dream of doing, if given the choice.

We have been raised to turn away from any awareness of this from an early age. Those we love and trust had that same upbringing. We follow this familiar path, eating the way our family and society eats, and the way our doctors, government, and other authorities encourage us to eat. Most of us continue this way, rather than daring to examine our food choices. To question our participation in this food system feels like a major act of rebellion, perhaps even radical. As much as we like to see ourselves as individualists, going against these deeply entrenched norms is not so easy.

Throughout history, there have been daring leaders who advocated for a vegetarian lifestyle, long before the word "vegan" was coined, before being plant-based was fashionable in Western cultures, and before there were so many critical reasons for shifting what we eat. Since early times, these compassionate advocates have promoted the ethical and health benefits of eating plants rather than animals. I find inspiration from these historical vegetarians, who included Pythagoras, Plutarch, Leonardo DaVinci, Leo Tolstoy, Mahatma Gandhi, Thomas Edison, Benjamin Franklin, Susan B. Anthony, George Bernard Shaw, Rosa Parks, and Albert Einstein.[36]

These vegetarian forerunners warned of the harm caused by our consumption of animals, and now the stakes are much higher. Our choice to ignore these warnings is leading to tragic results for our own well-being, the health of those we love, the animals we share this planet with, and the planet itself. It's imperative that we start to explore ways to change how we eat and how we live. It's time to let our compassion expand to all beings, including the animals that become commodities in our food system. And we also need to extend compassion toward ourselves, making choices that truly nurture our physical, mental, emotional, and spiritual well-being.

For those who are not yet vegan, this lifestyle may seem impossible. It may seem restrictive, depriving, or extreme. I certainly felt that way before I shifted to a vegetarian lifestyle and then later to a vegan one. For the first forty years of my life, I believed that meat and dairy were essential. To consider changing my lifestyle seemed overwhelming to me, especially without any role models or support. It took a series of steps to move into a plant-based lifestyle, starting with greater awareness that led me into action. Over time, my vegan path turned into a journey that was exciting and fulfilling. Although I don't generally consider myself to be a rebel (okay, maybe occasionally), I have embraced the opportunity to advocate for a more healthful, humane, and ecologically sound approach to what we eat and the food system that sustains all of us.

Some basic definitions

Before going further, here are some definitions to help clarify what veganism is, as well as *plant-based*, *vegan*, and *whole-food, plant-based* diets:

Veganism

"Veganism is a philosophy and way of living which seeks to exclude—as far as is possible and practicable—all forms of exploitation of, and cruelty to, animals for food, clothing, or any other purpose; and by extension, promotes the development and use of animal-free alternatives for the benefit of animals, humans, and the environment. In dietary terms, it denotes the practice of dispensing with all products derived wholly or partly from animals" (Definition from The Vegan Society, founded in 1944).[37]

Vegan (or plant-based) diet

Excludes all animal products (no meat, fish, dairy, eggs, or animal byproducts). Includes any foods from the plant kingdom: vegetables, greens, mushrooms, fruits, beans, lentils, tofu, tempeh, whole grains, nuts, and seeds. It may also include processed and prepared foods made from plant-sourced ingredients. (Note: Be aware that some sources may use the term *plant-based* to denote a *mostly*, but not exclusively, plant-sourced diet.)

Whole-food, plant-based diet

A plant-exclusive diet that primarily consists of unprocessed (or minimally processed) whole plant foods. Sugar, oils, and salt are often limited or may be eliminated entirely. Sometimes referred to as a "whole-food, vegan diet" to clarify that no animal products are included.

Vegetarian diet

Includes foods from the plant kingdom. Excludes meat, fish, and poultry, but may include dairy products or eggs.

The vegan path

Many people think of veganism as a diet, but it is really much more than that. Veganism was originally defined as a philosophy and way of living that seeks to avoid exploitation and cruelty toward animals through our food choices, as well as clothing and other purchases. With growing public awareness of the benefits of plant-based diets, people are drawn to veganism for a variety of reasons, including not only animal compassion and ethics, but also health, social justice, and the environment. When we enter the doorway to veganism for one of these reasons, we often discover the other benefits as well.

Although not a "diet" in the traditional way we think of the word, veganism does involve changing food habits, and that's something that many of us find challenging, at least initially. You may find it difficult to let go of the familiar cultural and social traditions. It may be hard to imagine breaking free from certain addictive foods. And it may feel overwhelming to step outside of the eating norms of society and your social circle. You may wonder, "How do I even do this vegan thing, anyway?" Especially if you don't have any role models to show you an accessible and achievable way to make the transition.

However, what many of us discover, once we start on the vegan path, is that there is a plethora of support to guide us in making this transition sustainably and enjoyably. We find that not only is a plant-based lifestyle doable, it's also delicious and satisfying. Rather than depriving, it is abundant. There are many styles of plant-based eating, many types of cuisine, and many pathways to starting a plant-powered lifestyle. Through the resources and inspirational stories that are offered in this book, you'll have the opportunity to discover the approach that works best for you.

Becoming vegan does not solve all problems, for yourself or for the world. However, for many it is part of a journey toward becoming more aware of how our actions impact the greater well-being of ourselves and the world—and toward being willing to make aligned choices. *The good news is: This is not an either-or choice. Caring for the greater good through eating plant-based has huge benefits for us as well.*

Becoming vegan is part of an awakening that has the potential to vastly improve your health and your overall mind-body-spirit wellness.

While there are many books on the physical health benefits of a plant-based lifestyle, fewer books describe the psychological, emotional, and spiritual alignment one may experience. In my surveys and interviews with vegans, many reported that their sense of integrating mind, body, and spirit was actually more fulfilling than any physical healing. Many described a sense of peace, fulfillment, and freedom that far outweighed any challenges of stepping out of old patterns into this new way of living.

Healing mind, body, and spirit

After reviewing hundreds of survey responses about vegans' emotional, social, and spiritual experiences, I found that seven transformative themes emerged. While not every participant reported experiencing *all* these themes, they emerged as the most common and most repeatedly referenced. These core themes were: values alignment, compassion, purpose, authentic fulfillment, meaningful relationships, health empowerment, and spiritual interconnectedness. I will describe each of these briefly next.

The courage to live by our deepest values

The vast majority of participants said that honoring their values through a vegan lifestyle was one of the most fulfilling and freeing aspects of being vegan. Many expressed the same feeling: "Finally I am truly living by my values of compassion and nonviolence." In Chapter Two, I discuss the benefits of identifying and living by our values, what blocks us from doing so, and how we can move toward greater fidelity with our core values.

Expanding our compassion

Most of us view compassion as an admirable quality, something to be nurtured. Yet, we may have blind spots when it comes to extending compassion toward those who are different from us. We also may limit our compassion to certain species of animals, excluding the animals in our food system. Chapter Three explores why cultivating compassion for *all beings* is good for us as well as for others, and how we can mindfully extend our circle of compassion to include ourselves, other humans, and all sentient beings.

Discovering greater meaning and purpose

Cultivating a sense of meaning and purpose is a driving force for many of us. Becoming vegan has the potential to increase our sense of purpose, as we realize that we have the power to create positive change in our world. Many of my research participants discovered ways to use their unique gifts and skills to raise awareness of the effects of our food choices and to create a kinder, healthier world. Chapter Four discusses the benefits of having meaning and purpose in our lives, how veganism contributes to our sense of meaning, and how to cultivate purpose.

Creating authentic fulfillment

Many vegans discover a deep sense of fulfillment in choosing to align with their vegan values. This fulfillment goes beyond the superficial, and often encompasses the whole range of emotional experience, from uplifting emotions such as contentment, happiness, and joy, to navigating difficult emotions like sadness, grief, and anger. Chapter Five shares how vegans find authentic well-being, and the benefits of plant-based nutrition for fueling better emotional health.

Building meaningful relationships

Relationships are a key aspect of our human experience. Many vegans find that in discovering meaningful values and purpose, they build authentic, satisfying connections with others who share these same convictions. Those who thrive as vegans also learn how to effectively communicate about their needs and values, while navigating conflicts and differences. Chapter Six dives into these topics so that we can strengthen meaningful connections with others.

Taking charge of our health

Chronic medical issues diminish our quality of life. Many vegans discover the powerful healing benefits of a plant-based diet and other lifestyle changes for managing and treating common degenerative diseases. This discovery brings something beyond physical healing; it brings a sense of empowerment, the realization that we have more control over our health and well-being than we ever knew. Chapter Seven shares the inspiring stories of vegans who have overcome debilitating illness to reclaim fulfilling and active lives. The chapter also shares resources for optimizing your health, fitness, and self-empowerment through plant-based nutrition and lifestyle medicine.

Discovering our interconnectedness with life

Once you are no longer eating animals, a new sense of awareness can emerge. Many of my vegan participants reported experiences of deepening spirituality, increased awe of the natural world, and a greater sense of their interconnection with all of nature and all life. Chapter Eight explores how we can cultivate self-transcendence and our sense of interconnectedness. I also discuss reasons why these experiences may, at least for some, go hand-in-hand with vegan values and lifestyle.

Bringing this all together

These seven transformative themes are supported by psychological, spiritual, and philosophical teachings as keys to a life that is rich, fulfilling, and meaningful. Becoming vegan doesn't guarantee that you will experience all these transformations. However, the experiences shared by my research participants demonstrate what is possible when we dare to question socially imposed "norms" that violate our own highest values and well-being, and instead listen to and follow our own deeper knowing, living (and eating) in ways that nourish body, mind, spirit, and the planet.

Wherever you are on your plant-based journey, whether just starting to eat more plants, or already a seasoned vegan, may this book be a companion on your path to inner clarity, to live your most healthy, fulfilling, and purposeful life. As we move on to Chapter Two, we will start by looking at the important role that our values play in living a life that is authentic and true, a life that brings peace, fulfillment, and well-being. How do we identify our core values? In what ways are we deviating from these values? And how do we make daily choices that truly honor our convictions? We'll take a closer look at these questions and hear personal stories that showcase the beautiful tapestry of values-aligned living.

PART TWO

THE PATH OF VEGAN TRANSFORMATION

CHAPTER 2

THE COURAGE TO LIVE YOUR VALUES

"You have just dined, and however scrupulously the slaughterhouse is concealed in the graceful distance of miles, there is complicity."

—**Ralph Waldo Emerson**

"Our complicity lies not in a direct infliction of violence but rather in our tacit agreement to look away and not to ask some very, very simple questions: Where does this meat come from and how did it get here?"

—**Timothy Pachirat**, author of *Every 12 Seconds: Industrialized Slaughter and the Politics of Sight* [1]

My awakening to vegan values

Animals have always had a special place in my life. As a child, I adored my pet cat, and I had a family of stuffed dogs that I played with and took with me everywhere. I didn't like to see any creature suffering, whatever their species. Even though I wasn't so fond of insects, I remember once rescuing a grasshopper that was floating on a lake, letting it jump on my raft so I could bring it back to shore.

Even though I loved animals, I thought that meat and dairy were necessary for my health and well-being. And I loved the meals my mother cooked, which generally involved some sort of meat, potatoes, and vegetables in a butter or cheese sauce, all washed down with a glass of milk.

I had little awareness of the animals that were bred, raised, and killed to be part of my daily meals. In fact, I rarely thought about the fact that meat comes from animals, or what was involved in the process that brought my food to me. If this thought did cross my mind, it was fleeting.

I did not see any other option. I had no idea what to eat if I stopped consuming meat and dairy products. These were staples in my diet, and they were convenient, easy, and comforting.

Program on PBS that opened my eyes

I had what I think of as my awakening a few weeks after my fortieth birthday, in December 2006. The news program I was watching featured a segment about workers in a meat processing plant. These workers, most of whom were immigrants, endured difficult working conditions and frequent occupational injuries due to the dangerous and repetitive nature of their work. They were coerced not to report their injuries but rather to continue working or face the threat of losing their jobs and income. Many were unable to obtain necessary medical treatment or recovery time because of the pressure to keep working and not take time off.

The program did not show any gory details of "meat processing," but I was deeply unsettled. Maybe it particularly struck me because, at the time, I was employed as a psychologist in a multidisciplinary pain management program, working with patients who suffered devastating emotional, physical, and financial impacts from work-related injuries. I witnessed the difficulties they faced with obtaining approvals for needed treatment and being allowed adequate time for recovery. It seemed to me that working in a meat processing plant (a.k.a. slaughterhouse) would be one of the most horrific jobs one could have.

As I felt empathy for the workers, it struck me that if I didn't like how the workers were treated, I would be appalled if I saw the slaughter process or how the animals were treated. For the first time in my life, I began to consider the systems that produced my food.

A door of possibility

Prior to watching this program, I had a rudimentary understanding that meat comes from animals and that they were killed in order to become what I called food. However, like many of us, I was very disconnected from this process. Although I grew up in small-town Iowa, surrounded by farms, I didn't know about factory farming. I knew only a few vegetarians or vegans, and I didn't understand why anyone would choose that lifestyle or what they would eat.

At the time I saw this program, I believed that plant-based eating would be far too difficult to implement personally—unless I became rich and could afford my own private chef. But now, with my new awareness, maintaining the status quo was no longer acceptable. Although the challenges of learning how to eat and cook using a plant-based approach seemed daunting, how could I support the cruelty wrought by animal agriculture and meat production? I knew that I no longer wanted to participate in industries that caused such destruction. I became determined to learn how to move toward a vegetarian lifestyle.

A door to new possibilities opened. The very next day after watching that program, I went to Barnes and Noble, bought my first vegetarian cookbook, and tried out a recipe for roasted red pepper, spinach, and artichoke lasagna. Because I was such a novice at cooking, I had to drive to a nearby K-Mart midway through the recipe to purchase appropriate pots and pans. The lasagna turned out to be delicious, full of vibrant colors and sumptuous flavors. I shared it with my boyfriend (now husband) and his family, and it got rave reviews. *Wow, who knew I could cook?*

I went on to read every book I could find in my local library about vegetarianism. I read about plant-based nutrition to make sure I was covering all my nutritional bases. I read about factory farming, how farmed animals were raised, and the conditions in which they lived. I also learned about the environmental impacts of industrialized animal agriculture. I found myself captivated—and horrified—by what I was learning.

At first, I still ate meat when it was served at social gatherings. However, at home I was eating vegetarian, and for the first time in my life, found that I enjoyed cooking. I realized that I had never liked handling meat, and always worried about it being cooked enough to avoid illnesses like salmonella. Now I began exploring new plant-based recipes, going to the health food store, and buying spices and condiments I had never used before. I expanded my food palette and found new freedom, joy, and creativity. Cooking ceased to be a chore, and instead became an enjoyable and meaning-filled adventure.

I continued reading about vegetarian ethics and lifestyle. As I came to really understand the way that farmed animals are bred and raised, the conditions they live in, and the eventual slaughter process, I knew I could not be part of this anymore. Watching videos and reading stories that showed the cruelty, suffering, and pain inherent in every step of the process, I was deeply distressed. I knew I needed to live and speak my truth: "*I'm no longer eating meat.*" I remember when I first said these words at a family dinner, feeling a mixture of anxiety at stepping out of expected norms, along with determination to live by my values even if it meant not "fitting in" socially.

I came to understand that despite what my upbringing and culture had taught me, I did not need animal flesh to thrive physically. In fact, research shows that a plant-based lifestyle can prevent and manage some of the most common degenerative diseases of our time, such as coronary heart disease, Type 2 diabetes, and even autoimmune disease.[2] My choice to stop eating meat was not only kinder to animals, but it was also better for my own health.

A deepening commitment

Over time, I came to see that all animal-sourced foods involve pain and cruelty. I realized that the living conditions for dairy cows and egg-laying hens are as cruel as those endured by animals raised for meat, and that at the end of their relatively short lives, they go through the same slaughter process. I started to limit dairy products and discovered that I was free of chronic seasonal allergies when I did so. I knew that becoming vegan was the right next step for me to honor my values more fully.

Still, it took time to fully move into veganism, working through my own inner challenges, shifting my mindset, and committing to this lifestyle change. Gradually, I broke through deep layers of emotional disconnection and social conditioning. At that point, there was no turning back.

When I stopped eating animals and embraced the bounty of the plant kingdom, I experienced positive changes I hadn't anticipated. Even though there were challenges along the way, once I committed, I felt a great inner peace. I felt freed, exhilarated, and awakened by this choice. I was free from past food habits and preferences that were not healthy for me. I was free from the subconscious weight of paying to kill sentient beings for my daily sustenance. I was free to find my voice and a deeper sense of purpose. I was free to be more authentically me.

I realized that making this choice was about more than my own ethics and personal health, even though these were important. It was about standing for a world of compassion, kindness, and sustainability. I came to see that so many things I cared about deeply were interconnected, that the daily choice of what we eat affects countless sentient beings, human health, the health of our planet, food availability, worker justice, and compassion and justice for all. Through embracing a vegan lifestyle and having the courage to defy social norms around what I ate and purchased, I discovered the peace that came with truly aligning my behaviors with my values. While, as an imperfect human in an imperfect world, I cannot fully avoid *all* harm to sentient beings, I can do my best to avoid and reduce harm and cruelty whenever possible.[3]

Being true to inner convictions and values

The peace and freedom that I found through living my vegan values is shared by many other vegans. When I asked my research respondents to select from a checklist all the ways that veganism has contributed to their emotional well-being, the top response, endorsed by 85 percent of participants, was, "Being true to my inner convictions and values." This concept also came up again and again in responses to my open-ended follow-up question, "In your own words, what are the most positive changes in your emotional and spiritual well-being associated with being vegan?" Survey respondents expressed that through living a vegan lifestyle, they felt aligned with core values, morals, and ethics that mattered deeply to them, as reflected in the sampling of responses here:

> "The most positive change in my emotional well being associated with being vegan: Staying in alignment with core values, knowing that I am making the best choices possible for myself, the animals, and the planet."

> "The most positive is the peace that comes with being in harmony with my core morals and values by choosing a more life-affirming way."

> "[I feel] greater internal peace and sense of harmony arising from living in a manner that more fully aligns with my values of compassion and respect for all."

"I adore that my life is making the least impact possible in a world where we are faced with constant decisions. I find peace that my lifestyle is positive for the animals, the environment, and my health."

"Knowing that I am living according to my values. I feel like I found something that connected a lot of dots for me . . . and a lot of causes that were always near to my heart."

"There is a weight off my shoulders to be no longer involved in animal cruelty—although I didn't know that weight was on my shoulders until it lifted."

Further, many participants found that aligning daily choices with vegan values led to a cascade of positive outcomes, including greater peace, confidence, integrity, satisfaction, and purpose, as shown in the survey responses here:

"Feeling aligned with my values gives me a sense of integrity and peace. Knowing I'm doing what I can to reduce suffering gives my life meaning."

"Living in alignment with my true inner values has given me greater purpose and an increased sense of peace."

"I feel aligned with my deepest values. Veganism is as natural and right for me as breathing, and I feel a deep sense of happiness to be living this way."

"I had no idea that clarifying my values through going vegan would help me get more comfortable sticking to my values in so many ways."

"Veganism is how I achieve a deep, ethical life, expanding my concern for others and myself on so many levels. . . I am living a life of meaningful values now. I feel like I'm doing what I came here to do in the larger scheme of life, that I'm finally living a life of meaning, contributing to something greater than myself."

"Knowing that I'm being true to my beliefs leads to inner peace and feeling more connected to Earth. I experience emotional well-being, knowing no animals are being harmed or exploited for my gain. Being able to run my businesses with purely vegan products means I'm still able to work within my values."

"I would say that the most positive changes I experienced in my emotional and spiritual well-being that resulted from going vegan stemmed from finally aligning my values with my actions. After eating animal products for 35 years, the day I chose to commit to this lifestyle released a huge load of shame, grief, and inner conflict that I had experienced up till then when eating animals."

"Being vegan has allowed me to align with my highest values and be at complete happiness, peace, and joy in my life. I love where I am now that I have regained my health, and I'm living the compassionate life that I should have always been living. I am much more at peace with myself, knowing that I am not participating in cruelty to animals. This gives me a profound sense of peace that I never knew before."

What are values and why do they matter?

The Oxford Languages Dictionary defines *values* as: "A person's principles or standards of behavior; one's judgment of what is important in life."

Our core values are basic and fundamental beliefs that guide our attitudes and choices. They help us to determine what is important to us and how to act accordingly. Values are our moral compass. They describe the personal qualities we choose to embody and the kind of person we want to be. They guide how we treat ourselves and others and show us how to be authentic, so that we act in ways that reflect what really matters to us. Values play a key role in forming our sense of identity.

Knowing what your values are, what you believe, and what matters to you can help you to make decisions that are best for you. We tend to be healthier psychologically when our thoughts, feelings, and goals are in alignment with our values. As my research participants noted, living in alignment with our values can lead to greater fulfillment, self-worth, and sense of purpose. And yet many of us haven't taken the time to reflect on or define our core values, much less determine if we are living in alignment with them.

When we are young, our values are shaped by our upbringing and our culture. As adults, we may or may not have taken the time to see if these values suit us, and if we are living in ways that reflect what truly matters to us. In addition, it can take courage to follow our values when they require us to stand up to peer pressure or societal expectations. In my many years working as a psychotherapist, I have found that being out of touch (and out of sync) with our values is a major contributor to the emotional malaise and existential distress that many of us face.

What happens when we do not live in alignment with our values?

When we act in ways that do not match our values, and we become aware of this inner inconsistency, we may experience what is called *cognitive dissonance*. This concept was introduced in 1957 by Leon Festinger, a psychologist.[4] Cognitive dissonance is the mental discomfort that comes from holding two or more conflicting beliefs, attitudes, or values, or behaving in ways that are not in sync with our personal values. This misalignment between our beliefs and behaviors can contribute to an inner conflict that is uncomfortable or downright distressing.

The tension and stress of cognitive dissonance is heightened depending on the *level* of disparity between our beliefs and actions, and how much the conflicting beliefs or values *matter* to us. It can be especially distressing when we are out of alignment with values that are central to our moral compass or our identity. When we act against our core principles, we may feel shame or guilt, or inwardly question our "goodness" or integrity.

How do we cope with cognitive dissonance?

We may handle this discomfort by justifying, rationalizing, or explaining away the inner conflict between our beliefs and behaviors. We may even change our beliefs or perceptions so that we no longer feel the inner conflict. For example, someone who has tried to quit smoking but then relapses might minimize the risks of cigarette smoking or question the benefits of quitting. They may then come up with stories that seem to support this, to help lessen any discomfort that comes with not aligning their behavior with their goal.

This inner dissonance may play out with a variety of values we hold. Some examples include desiring to be healthy, but eating unhealthy food; wanting to be physically fit, but not exercising; wishing to be kind and patient, but speaking or acting unkindly to others; or caring about the environment, but continuing to purchase items in single-use plastic containers.

The discomfort of cognitive dissonance usually leads to one of the following choices: We change our *behaviors* so that they better match our values, or we alter our *perceptions* to lessen the inner conflict and associated discomfort. This can occur through changing our values so that they match our behaviors, or perhaps more commonly, through shifting our perceptions to obscure any contradictions between our values and behaviors. We also may compartmentalize our behavior to avoid awareness of these contradictions.

How does this relate to veganism?

Many of us adore dogs and cats. We cherish them as companions and beloved family members. We buy special food for them, spend time and money on their care, and let them sleep next to us (or in their own special bed). When our pets die, we are heartbroken. An indicator of how important they are to us is the money that we spend on them. According to the American Pet Products Association, Americans spent $136.8 billion on their pets in 2022.[5]

We also appreciate the birds who populate our bird feeders and many of us are fascinated by wildlife. Most of us have compassion for animals and abhor seeing them experience cruelty, suffering, or neglect. This concern is reflected in our financial support to groups who protect animals; Americans donate over $1 billion to animal welfare groups each year.[6]

However, we are conditioned from a young age to view farmed animals who are raised for meat differently from other animals. As Colleen Patrick-Goudreau points out in her book *The Joyful Vegan*, we are taught to view chickadees as *friends* (and worthy of admiring, helping, and saving) and chickens as *dinner*.[7] Similarly, many of us view pigs, cows, sheep, goats, and other farmed animals differently than dogs or cats, even though they, too, are sentient beings.

Currently, we are eating more animals than at any other time in human history. Over ninety billion land animals are slaughtered globally per year, ten billion each year in the United States alone.[8] When you consider our consumption of fish and other sea creatures, these numbers are in the trillions. According to a 2020 statistic, the average American consumes 264 pounds of meat per year.[9] The amount of meat consumed annually by Americans has increased by 35 to 40 percent over the past sixty years.[10]

Currently, America is one of the top consumers of meat compared to other countries. However, as industrialization—supported by government subsidies to the meat industry—increases the production and availability of meat globally, meat consumption is growing in other countries as well, including those whose diets were traditionally more plant based.[11]

And yet, even with the rising global consumption of meat, most of us desire humane treatment for animals. One doesn't have to identify as an "animal lover" to abhor cruelty and unnecessary suffering. A 2015 national poll conducted by HuffPost/YouGov found that 86 percent of meat-eating Americans say it's important that farmed animals are treated humanely. This concern for the humane treatment of animals was shown across political party affiliation, income, sex, and race.[12]

How do we make sense of this disconnect between our concern for the well-being of animals and the reality that billions of them are bred, raised, and slaughtered each year for human consumption in ways that would horrify the average person if they looked more closely? Paul McCartney is noted for saying, "If slaughterhouses had glass walls, everyone would be vegetarian." This suggests that most people are not aware of the inhumane conditions associated with meat production, and that if they were, they would not participate.

However, even though the internet gives us increased access to videos and information that show what happens in factory farms and slaughterhouses,[13] most of us never seek out this footage or try to learn what happens to the animals we think of as "meat."[14] Why is this? How do we understand our collective cognitive dissonance? Most of us care about animals, and yet we routinely pay industries to treat them inhumanely and kill them for our food. Next, I discuss some factors that play a role in this disconnect.

Carnism

Why do we love dogs and cats, but eat pigs, cows, chickens, and turkeys? This was the question that social psychologist Melanie Joy, Ph.D., author of the ground-breaking book *Why We Love Dogs, Eat Pigs, and Wear Cows*, explored as part of her doctoral research. Joy, who has extensively studied the psychology of violence and injustice, sought to better understand why people extend compassion to some species of animals, while being indifferent to the welfare of other species.

When exploring questions around why we eat pigs and not dogs with her students and research participants, often the answers Joy received were along the lines of, "I don't know. I never thought about it. I guess, because it's just the way things are." Joy goes on to say, "Take a moment to consider this statement. Really think about it. We send one species to the butcher and give our love and kindness to another apparently for no reason other than because *it's the way things are.*"[15]

The key underlying cause of this widespread disconnect is *carnism*, a term that Joy coined to describe the invisible ideology that surrounds the eating of meat. Carnism is defined as "the belief system that conditions us to eat certain animals."[16] Joy explains that because carnism is invisible, often we don't realize that eating animals is a choice rather than a given. We don't think about why we eat certain animals and not others, or why we eat animals at all. When a practice such as meat-eating is so entrenched, so longstanding and prevalent, we don't see that there is a belief system and choice involved. We think "it's just the way things are."

Yet, because most of us care deeply for animals and have at least some awareness of the suffering of farmed animals, we may struggle with an inner conflict, a form of cognitive dissonance (there's that term again). As discussed earlier, there are a few primary ways to reduce our cognitive dissonance: we can change our behaviors to match our values, we can change our values, or we can change our perceptions about our existing behaviors (so they no longer seem to conflict with our values).

When it comes to eating animals, we can cope with our inner conflict by changing our behavior: reducing our meat intake or becoming vegetarian or vegan. Those of us not ready or willing to alter our meat consumption may instead change our perceptions to reduce any sense of inner conflict. Joy's research found that we mount a variety of psychological defenses to distance ourselves from discomfort about eating animals. For example: denial, avoidance, minimalization, compartmentalization, rationalization, justification, and dissociation.

The system of carnism is perpetuated by what Joy calls the *Three Ns of Justification*: meat-eating is portrayed by authorities, institutions, mass media, and the culture at large as *"normal, natural, and necessary."* Joy explains, "The Three Ns are so ingrained in our social consciousness that they guide our actions without our even having to think about them."[17] We are led to believe this is the way things have always been and the way they are meant to be. However, many atrocities and injustices throughout history, atrocities that we now condemn, were once rationalized as *normal, natural, and necessary.*[18]

We are taught from a young age that we need to consume meat and dairy for our health and survival. As we go through life, this message continues to be perpetuated by authority figures like teachers, parents, and health professionals, who were all raised with the same messages. We don't see that we have a choice to stop eating animals.

However, when we look more closely at the vast number of plant-based, vegan, and vegetarian people who have thrived with a meat-free diet, we have to ask—Is it true that eating meat is *necessary*? When we look at the horrific and inhumane conditions for farmed animals and what's involved in the slaughter process, we have to ask—Is it true that this is *natural*? We might also ask—Is this truly *normal*? The practices around breeding and killing animals for meat may be so commonplace that they have become normalized. However, norms are not absolute truths, but are instead socially constructed. That is, norms are shaped by our interactions with others and by what is culturally accepted. When we listen to our own inner compass, we may decide that we do not want to contribute to or support some of the things that are considered "normal" in society.

Speciesism

While there is increasing awareness of the prejudices and discrimination associated with entrenched ideologies such as *racism* and *sexism* in our culture, many of us are less aware of *speciesism*. Speciesism is the assumption of human superiority over other animals, and the prejudice and discrimination against certain beings based on their species. This ideology leads us to perceive some beings (humans and certain species of animals) as more valuable, deserving of greater rights and moral consideration than other species. This inherent speciesism allows us to value and care for some animals while disregarding the well-being of others. The speciesism that drives many of our decisions and choices is often invisible to us.

The meat paradox

This inner conflict between our caring for animals and yet eating a diet that contributes to the suffering and death of many animals has been called the *meat paradox*. This term was used by Dr. Steve Loughnan and his colleagues to describe the paradox of "how we are able to love animals and love eating animals."[19] There has been a significant amount of research and discussion on this topic, examining the evolution and impact of this inner conflict, as well as strategies people utilize to lessen their dissonance or discomfort.[20]

One of the ways that we lessen the inner conflict between meat eating and our desire to not harm animals is through forming negative perceptions of certain species of animals. Studies have found that people rate animals categorized as "food" as being less capable of suffering and less worthy of moral concern. In addition, the very act of eating meat may increase these justifications. Research participants who were asked to consume meat as part of a study rated cows as less capable of suffering and having lesser minds, compared to participants who were asked to consume plant foods.[21]

Other strategies that are used to reduce discomfort about meat eating include denying the harm to farmed animals, discrediting sources that share information on the harms of meat-eating, or holding biased negative views of those who don't eat meat. An additional strategy is to actively avoid situations or information that would cause uneasiness about eating meat.[22]

What contributes to the meat paradox?

There are numerous personal and social factors that may play into why we continue to eat meat, even when it conflicts with our ethical values. For example:

1. **The invisibility of factory farms and slaughterhouses**. Many of us are ignorant of the treatment of farmed animals. Most of the large-scale, industrialized factory farms are out of sight in rural areas. Because we never see these operations, we are distanced from the process by which animals are bred, raised, and slaughtered.

2. **Meat industry packaging and terminology**. The terms used to describe meat, and the way that meat is packaged and advertised,

further distances us from the animal that the meat comes from. For example, the sterile-looking packages we see at the deli counter or in the meat aisle seem far removed from their animal source. In addition, many of the terms used to label cuts of meat (e.g., calling cow flesh "beef" or "steak," and pig flesh "bacon," "pork," or "ham") may make them more appealing to consumers and camouflage the realities of the animal slaughter necessary to produce them. When the animal source of meat or dairy products *is* mentioned in advertising or packaging, it is often falsely portrayed as "happy," "humane," or "natural."

3. **Conflicting messages about nutrition**. We receive confusing and often contradictory information about health, nutrition, and diet through the media, government, schools, and healthcare professionals. These messages lead us to believe that we need meat in order to be healthy, even though a substantial body of research indicates that plant-based diets are nutritious and can prevent, manage, and even reverse many common medical conditions. In fact, the Position Paper of the American Dietetic Association states that "appropriately planned vegetarian diets, including total vegetarian or vegan diets, are healthful, nutritionally adequate, and may provide health benefits in the prevention and treatment of certain diseases."[23]

4. **Agribusiness advertising**. Large agricultural corporations spend vast sums of money on advertising to convince us of the benefits and necessity of meat and dairy products. As Zoe Weil, Ph.D., co-founder and president of the Institute for Humane Education, eloquently states, "Profit-driven companies manipulate us to want their products, foods, and services, even if we have no need for them; even if they are unhealthy; even if they use up our precious time and cost us money; even if their production is cruel, unjust, or destructive . . . In other words, our deepest values become eclipsed by manufactured desires."[24]

5. **Food patterns and cravings**. Our food preferences, habits, and addictions can make it difficult to change our eating patterns. Many people enjoy the taste of meat, cheese, and other animal products.[25] On top of that, dairy foods (especially cheese) are known to be addictive,

in part because of the casomorphins they contain. Casomorphins are a morphine-like compound found in mothers' milk that help to calm and soothe their nursing babies. These casomorphins are most highly concentrated in cheese. This may be part of the reason why many people find animal-based cheese so hard to give up![26]

In addition, we are biologically wired to crave foods high in salt, fat, and sugar. Food producers are aware of this and capitalize on it when they create processed foods and snacks. This includes many of the meat and dairy products that people enjoy. Think about gourmet cheese, sweetened café lattes, pepperoni and cheese pizza, or hamburgers. The flavorings, ingredients, and condiments that make these products tasty are usually packed with a hefty dose of salt, fat, and/or sugar. Research shows that the more we eat these types of foods, the more we crave them.[27]

6. **Family and social traditions**. Meat-eating is tied to family, social, and cultural customs, and for many people it can be emotionally (and socially) difficult to break away from these norms and traditions. We may feel a strong emotional attachment to foods that were part of our upbringing and our early memories of special times with family and loved ones. In addition, it takes courage and effort to step out of the socially approved practice of eating meat and to be different from those around us.

7. **Emotional eating**. Some of us struggle with personal issues around eating that make dietary changes an especially emotionally charged matter. These struggles may range from comfort eating to soothe emotions to severe eating disorders such as bulimia, anorexia, or binge eating. Those with severe eating disorders or addictions may need professional help to recover; however, most healthcare professionals and recovery programs are not attuned to or trained in the benefits of healthy plant-based nutrition as part of this recovery.

As you think about the impacts of carnism and speciesism in your own experience, I invite you to reflect: Why do so many of us view the lives of dogs, cats, and humans as valuable, while not holding the same regard for a chicken, pig, cow, or lobster? What have you learned that helps you make sense of this?

Benefits of aligning with vegan values

For many vegans, there is an awakening that leads them to shift to a vegan lifestyle, whether it is something they learned, a personal health crisis, or an unexpected experience that opened their eyes. For some people that shift happens overnight. For others, it's a lengthier process that emerges over time. Whether the change was immediate or took time to unfold, my research participants found that aligning with their values through a vegan lifestyle brought a cascade of positive inner changes, such as greater peace, confidence, integrity, freedom, fulfillment, meaning, and harmony.

They were also freed from the previously unrecognized inner conflict around eating meat. As expressed by one survey participant, "I no longer have to deal with the cognitive dissonance of saying 'I love animals' while paying to abuse them." Another said, "There is an incredible sense of confidence and inner peace knowing that you are living in line with your true values. I have never felt so healthy and true to myself. This feels like I am my authentic self for the first time in my life."

Vegan living is an embodied expression of values such as physical health, care for our planet, nonviolence, and compassion for all sentient beings. Nancy Arenas is a vegan whose story demonstrates the transformative power of aligning with vegan values. Like many vegans, she had an unexpected awakening that made her realize the ethical impact of her food choices. Her own healing experience led her to dedicate her life to helping others awaken to the benefits of a vegan lifestyle.

Nancy A.'s story

Nancy Arenas is the host of the Vegan Pulse podcast, publisher of *New Mexico Vegan Magazine*, and founder and organizer of Red & Green Veg Fest of Albuquerque.[28] While she is an active vegan advocate now, this was something she couldn't have imagined years ago. Like many of us, she ate a typical American diet for most of her life and had not given thought to the animals that composed much of this diet.

Her vegan journey began around 2013, after a visit from an old friend from college. He had been vegan for years, and she thought he was going to be proud of her because she had recently become vegetarian. She said, "I waited for the right moment and said, 'Guess what? I'm vegetarian.' I was waiting for him to say, 'Atta girl!' or give me a big pat on the back. But it really didn't come."

Nancy expressed to her friend that she was disappointed by his tepid response. He responded, "Well, being vegetarian is better." Nancy asked, "What do you mean *better*?" And her friend explained, "It's better than you were eating before. But you're not vegan." Nancy realized that she didn't understand what he meant. She asked what was the difference between vegetarian and vegan? He went on to explain that she was still regularly drinking milk and eating cheese, and that this contributed to suffering as well. He shared with her the exploitation and horrific conditions that dairy cows experience.

Nancy said, "Right then and there, it was like a spark. I said, 'Okay, I'm vegan'—just like that." She described herself as someone who has always been spiritual, who has tried to live by a "do no harm" philosophy since she was very young. She added, "In spite of that, I had never made the connection between animals and eating and the harm this does. I thought, 'I don't want to harm anything or anyone. It makes sense to go vegan.'"

Becoming vegan was a big change for Nancy. She loved cheese and milk, and previously had believed they were necessary for good health. She added, "I even did one of those milk mustache commercials back in the 1980s. The ones that go 'Got milk?' We're taught from the commercials that 'milk does a body good' and that milk gives us strong bones. Right? Which I've since learned is not the truth." Despite loving cheese and being in a milk commercial, she decided, "I'm going vegan because I don't want to participate in the torture or harm of animals."

Nancy emphasized, "I didn't care about the health aspect of being vegan. I did it solely for the animals." However, she had suffered from fibromyalgia for years, with daily pain levels of seven out of ten. She did not see the connection between her pain and her diet, but to her surprise, exactly one month after becoming vegan, she woke up with no pain. She shared her reaction to this sudden and unexpected pain relief:

I thought, "Something's wrong, because I'm not feeling the pain I usually feel." I later realized that it was because I let go of the milk and other animal products. I guess I had flushed all these things out of my system. I'm not a doctor, so I don't know for sure. But my migraines disappeared. My vertigo went away. The joint swelling, bursitis, and most importantly, the fibromyalgia all went away. My sensitive stomach also improved. And at first, I couldn't comprehend what happened. It really was an awakening for me. At that moment, I said, "Can you imagine that? Because I was kind to the animals, the Universe decided to be kind to me."

And I realized, the doctors—or corporations—they aren't telling anyone, "Hey, why don't you switch to a plant-based diet and see if you get relief from some of these physical symptoms?"

Nancy indicated that she went through different stages as she adapted to her vegan lifestyle. "At first, I thought I had to have a meat substitute . . . Over time I became more of a whole-food, plant-based eater." She learned that vegetables, fruits, beans, and grains could provide the protein and other nutrients she needed. She added that she also went through different emotional stages. "When I first went vegan, I felt really good because I was no longer hurting animals." But then she went through a phase of being frustrated by the lack of vegan options available in her grocery store and local restaurants. She said:

Eventually, after being angry and frustrated about all this, I decided to get educated instead and to educate others. I started to educate the restaurants. When they said that they didn't have anything vegan on the menu, I would say, "Okay, you have rice, does it have anything in it that has animal products? No? Okay, that's vegan. And then you have beans and vegetables." We would go down the list, and I'd show them that they did have vegan options. I wanted to make up for the lost time, all those years I was supporting animal torture. I thought, What can I do to help educate others, to bring veganism forth?

In 2015, I decided to create an online magazine, *New Mexico Vegan Magazine*, which shares stories and inspiration about veganism . . . I have a history of being an event coordinator, so I decided to create a local Veg Fest in Albuquerque, and it's been going strong. I kept it alive during COVID by making it virtual. That had its own positives, because I could invite people who would otherwise not have been able to come and speak at it. I've had wonderful speakers like Carol Adams, Seb Alex, Sailesh Rao, Will Tuttle, Jane Velez-Mitchell, and Dr. Joel Kahn . . . For me, personally, what I got out of it was connecting people and forwarding veganism.

I tried to live by "do no harm" and be the peace child, growing up in New York in the 1970s. I thought I was such a big activist back then, you know, standing for peace, no war, and all this, and then, when I went vegan, I truly understood. "Wow, now I am really living that." I realized that before, I was just kind of scratching the surface of it . . . When you truly align yourself, in your every day, from the moment you get up to the moment you lay down, you realize, "I really am living this, I am really being my message."

When you make that connection, you start looking at everything differently. And then you realize that veganism is about connecting with everything. It's not just the diet, it's a whole lot of things . . . I have always been an animal lover, but mainly a dog lover. Now since I've been vegan, when I go into my yard, I've had the greatest experiences, because I was actually paying attention. There's a difference between seeing and actually seeing.

That's the thing about awakening—you thought you were already there. Throughout my life, I have always enjoyed the sunsets, the flowers, the colors, and the trees. But now everything has a whole new different look to it, and a different sound to it. It's like when I had LASIK surgery years ago . . . You know, fifteen minutes after I had LASIK, I thought I could see—and then, an hour later, I could actually see what I had been missing.

Nancy indicated that she has found additional avenues for sharing her passion for veganism. She taught a vegan cooking class at her local natural food store. She recalled that these classes were filled to "standing room only" with people who wanted to learn how to move toward a plant-based lifestyle.

After the COVID-19 pandemic started in 2020, when she couldn't do the cooking classes, she began a podcast called the *Vegan Pulse*, interviewing vegans from across the globe on topics such as cruelty-free fashion, vegan cooking, nutrition, and health. She added, "Promoting veganism has become my passion, not only because of animal suffering, but because people are not being told that they could feel better—and I think that's just not right."

Becoming vegan has also helped her emotionally. "I used to struggle with depression. And I tried in my own ways to get that under control, through martial arts and Buddhism meditation." She stated that since becoming vegan, she doesn't experience these mood fluctuations anymore. "If I do feel down, it's because something depressing is happening." She went on to add, "Sometimes my heart breaks when I think of animal suffering. But I think of a saying from Buddhism: 'Suffer what there is to suffer and celebrate what there is to celebrate and keep on.' I remind myself that the only way that we can stop this is if I get up, keep moving forward, and keep trying to bring it to the forefront."

When asked what it was like to do the podcast and public speaking about veganism, she said, "It's not so much that I'm brave, it's that this is something that needs to change. Instead of thinking about my fear, I think about the animals." In expanding on this, Nancy commented:

I try to explain to people that veganism truly is a social justice issue, because it's not just the animals and our health, it's about our planet and the future of our children. It has racial impacts, too, because slaughterhouses and factory farms have many employees who are minorities, and these workers become sick from the fumes and the manure that they spray. It's time to open up our minds . . . The planet is screaming, "Go vegan or die." I have a grandson who I would love to be able to see grow up in a world he can enjoy. Not a world where the water is polluted, where we can't breathe the air. It's kind of naive to think that veganism is about a diet. It affects us all.

I never thought I was going to be a vegan advocate when I turned vegan. I never really thought, "Oh, I'm going to be doing all this stuff to promote veganism." But then again, I never thought that my body was going to be healed when I went vegan. I was just trying to be kind to the animals. And when that kindness came back to me, I thought perhaps it was time to spread the joy to others as well, so that they could experience it too. We all really need to think about being more compassionate, changing our ways. We need to go vegan. We need to go to a whole-food, plant-based diet . . . We need to stop and think for a second and make a new world . . . One that is for everybody.

I was deeply moved by Nancy's story and her courage, the way she lives her values in everyday life, and the way she brings her values forth to help other people, animals, and the planet. She does all this while working in her regular full-time job! She expressed that her passion for veganism and creating a more compassionate world gives her the energy to take on the duties of her podcast, magazine, and local Veg Fest.

In some ways, the positive impact of aligning with vegan ethics and values was one of the most surprising findings of my research. When we think about what leads to a healthier and more fulfilling life, values alignment isn't top on the list for many of us. It can be challenging to pause and recognize our values in a frenetic world where we are distracted by so many competing stimuli and demands. It takes courage to honor our convictions, especially when doing so goes against what is comfortable, easy, or socially accepted. When you move toward a vegan lifestyle, you become one of the early adopters of what will eventually be seen as the ethical and just way to live. As expressed by vegan activist John Oberg, "One day, future generations will look back and say, 'I can't believe they used to eat animals.'"[29]

Action Steps

What follows are some reflections and action steps to help you discover your core values. You may want to create a journal for writing out your responses and reflections. Consider: How would moving toward a plant-based, vegetarian, or vegan lifestyle help you to be more in sync with your deepest values? If you are already plant-based or vegan, what additional steps would bring you into even greater alignment with your values?

- **Reflection question:** *What are your core values?* If you are not sure, go through the following reflections to help you identify them. Write your responses in your journal:
  o What matters most to you? What do you want in life, for yourself and for others?
  o Consider past experiences when you were being most true to yourself or when you felt most authentic. What values were represented in these experiences?

o Consider times that you were most proud of yourself. What made you feel that way? What qualities and values did you exhibit?

o Consider the times that you felt most at peace. What was it about those experiences that brought peace? What do you most value about these experiences?

o What kind of person do you aspire to be? What qualities do you want to be known for?

o Consider the traits of people you highly respect. What values do they demonstrate? What causes do they stand for?

o What kind of world do you want to see? What qualities and values would make this world a better place?

- **Based on these reflections, write a list of your core values.** After making your list, narrow it down to your top three to five values. Your values can reflect personal qualities, such as honesty, compassion, integrity, and dependability. They can also reflect issues that you care about deeply, such as the environment, spirituality, or social justice.

- **What do each of your top values mean to you?** How do they show up in your life? When have you felt in alignment with them? When have you felt out of alignment?

- **Identify one action for each of your top values**, in order to live this value more fully and consistently.

- **How do your purchasing choices fit with your values?** Most of us are unaware of the connections between our values and what we consume, since we rarely see the process by which our food or other items are produced. This is by design, since corporations know that most of us would not want to buy items whose production involved injustice toward workers, violence toward animals, or harm to the environment. To know whether our food or other items we purchase are truly humane, sustainable, and cruelty-free, we will likely need to do some research. Consider checking out the websites of the Environmental Working Group (EWG), People for the Ethical Treatment of Animals (PETA), Humane Society of the United States (HSUS), or other organizations that have guides to assess the ethical and environmental impact of various products and industries.

- **Consider the definition of *veganism* offered by The Vegan Society:** "Veganism is a way of living that seeks to exclude, as far as possible and practicable, all forms of exploitation of, and cruelty to, animals for food, clothing and any other purpose." How does this description of veganism fit with your own core values? To what degree are you living by this? What is one step that you can take toward greater alignment?

Discovering and living our values—and recognizing the ways that the vested interests of society, corporations, or authorities seek to disconnect us—can be part of a path to greater fulfillment, authenticity, and freedom. One of the values that is essential to healthy relationships, our personal fulfillment, and the well-being of our world is compassion. The next chapter explores the topic of compassion, how it relates to veganism, and why it is beneficial for our thriving as individuals, as well as the thriving of the larger ecosystems in which we reside.

CHAPTER 3

EXPAND YOUR CIRCLE OF COMPASSION

"If you want others to be happy, practice compassion. If you want to be happy, practice compassion."

—The Dalai Lama

"Compassion towards animals is so natural to us that only through conditioning could we become callous toward their suffering and death."

—Leo Tolstoy

"Our task must be to free ourselves from this prison by widening our circle of compassion to embrace all living beings and all of nature."

—Albert Einstein

Compassion is a core value for many of us. In fact, we are wired for compassion and empathy. Despite all the negative events in the news that reflect the uncaring aspects of humanity, compassion for others is part of our biological and psychological make-up.[1] Science shows that we have neurobiological systems that cause us to instinctively seek to alleviate others' suffering.[2] From an evolutionary standpoint, compassion appears to be essential to our survival. Charles Darwin argued that concern and sympathy for others is our strongest human instinct, often even stronger than self-interest.[3]

And yet, even though compassion is part of our human nature, and is one of our core values, many of us compartmentalize how our compassion is expressed. We may be compassionate toward certain people and certain situations, but disregard and lack empathy for others. This shows up in the polarization, division, and disconnection that is so prevalent in our society today.

This compartmentalization of our compassion is also evidenced in our treatment of animals. As highlighted in Chapter Two, even though compassion and concern for the well-being of animals is a core value for many of us, by and large, we have centered our compassion and care toward certain species of animals, such as pets and "desirable" wildlife, while disregarding and dismissing the treatment of animals in factory farming, research, entertainment, and other industries that use and exploit animals.

I consider myself a highly empathic person, but until that fateful day when I saw the PBS program about meat processing plants (as described in previous chapters), I was blind to what happened to the animals who became my food. Because of my social and cultural conditioning, along with the cunning tactics of the meat and dairy industries, I was blocked from seeing the plight of farmed animals and from holding compassion for them. I simply didn't know—and part of me didn't *want* to see or know. And then, after a series of priming events (including that news program), my eyes finally were opened, along with my compassion.

I'll never forget reading *Diet for a New America* early in my veg journey.[4] As the author, John Robbins, described the conditions in which farmed animals lived, the slaughter process, and the health and environmental consequences of animal agriculture, I was horrified. I wondered, "How could I not have known this before?" When I saw pictures of factory farms and learned about the crowded, confined, filthy conditions that farmed animals were raised in, the painful procedures they underwent, and the violence and trauma of the slaughter process, my compassion compelled me to commit to a meat-free lifestyle.

My heightened awareness of the plight of farmed animals has caused me emotional distress—especially when I acknowledge the scope of suffering caused by animal agriculture. It can be painful to connect with this suffering, because at times it feels like there's not enough that I can do to help alleviate it. And yet, awakening my compassion has brought so much that is positive. I've found that nurturing my compassion is key to being true to myself and my values, and to becoming a better human.

Many vegans report an awakening of compassion and empathy as part of their vegan experience; this was a core theme that emerged through my research interviews and surveys. When asked about the ways that veganism has enhanced their emotional well-being, "deeper empathy and compassion" was endorsed by over 75 percent of participants. As one participant stated, "I didn't [initially] go vegan for the animals, but on my plant-based journey, I have been surprised by how my compassion for other living creatures has increased."

Another expressed, "I've found great solace in living in alignment with my values of compassion to all vulnerable others. I've become my best self through empathy. To ease another's suffering, and better yet, to help prevent it entirely, is the best way to live." In awakening compassion for all beings, we become more aware of suffering, which can be painful, but we also have the potential to experience greater alignment, fulfillment, and humanity as we make positive changes that lessen harm.

Understanding compassion and empathy

In seeking to better understand the role of compassion and empathy in our lives, it may be helpful to define each of these. They are often used interchangeably, and while they are related to one another, they are not one and the same. Merriam-Webster's Dictionary defines *empathy* as "the action of understanding, being aware of, being sensitive to, and vicariously experiencing the feelings, thoughts, and experience of another" without having these be fully or explicitly communicated. *Compassion* takes empathy a step further; it is the "sympathetic consciousness of others' distress together with a desire to alleviate it."[5]

An article in *Greater Good Magazine* elaborates, stating "Compassion literally means 'to suffer together.'" The article explains the connection between empathy and compassion: "While empathy refers more generally to our ability to take the perspective and feel the emotions of another person, compassion is when those feelings and thoughts include the desire to help."[6]

Daniel Goleman, author of *Emotional Intelligence*, states that empathy is a key component of emotional intelligence, along with self-awareness, self-regulation, motivation, and social skills.[7] Goleman described three types of empathy: cognitive empathy (taking the perspective of the other), emotional empathy (feeling with the other), and compassionate empathy (sensing what the other needs and being moved to help). Amy Wilson, author of the book *Empathy for Change*, argues that empathy must include all three of these elements to be effective in creating positive change for a better world.[8]

Thus, empathy is an important bridge for recognizing and feeling another's suffering or distress, while compassion leads us to take action to alleviate the other's suffering when possible. The importance of compassion as an essential ethical principle and practice has long been advocated by humanitarian and spiritual leaders. Karen Armstrong, expert on comparative religions and TED prize winner in 2008, argues that compassion "lies at the heart of all truly religious and ethical systems."[9]

Wired for compassion

Neuroscientists have found that there is a biological basis for our experience of empathy and compassion. Dacher Keltner, Ph.D., author of *Born to Be Good: The Science of a Meaningful Life*, notes that when we witness someone suffering, our own pain centers are also activated, along with our amygdala, which processes emotions and detects potential dangers. However, as we move from empathy into compassion, this also engages parts of the brain associated with nurturing. Keltner states, "We don't just see suffering as a threat. We also instinctively want to alleviate that suffering through nurturance."[10]

Responding to another's suffering additionally stimulates the vagus nerve, which slows our heart rate, along with innervating communication systems that convey caring and warmth through our gaze and vocalizations. The vagus nerve, part of our parasympathetic nervous system, impacts numerous bodily functions, such as digestion, heart rate, and immune function. In studies, individuals with a stronger vagal response showed increased helpfulness and expressed a greater sense of connection and common humanity with diverse groups.[11]

While compassion starts with an empathic recognition of another's feelings or experience, empathy and compassion appear to follow different neural pathways. Social neuroscience researchers Tania Singer and Olga Klimecki note that our empathic awareness of another's suffering can result in one of two reactions: 1) *empathic distress*, in which we strongly identify with the other's suffering and have difficulties differentiating our self from the other, or 2) *empathic concern*, also referred to as *compassion*. Empathic distress creates an aversive response, including a desire to withdraw from the situation to lessen overwhelming negative feelings. Chronic empathic distress can lead to burnout and poor health over time. In contrast, empathic concern or compassion is characterized by warmth and care for the other, along with a desire to help.[12]

Compassionate behaviors make us feel good. Keltner notes, "When we give to others, or act cooperatively, reward centers in the brain (such as the nucleus accumbens, a region dense with dopamine receptors) hum with activity."[13] Research has shown that learning to strengthen compassion is associated with increased resilience and positive health outcomes.[14]

Although compassion fatigue is a well-known term for describing the experience of caregivers and caring professionals who chronically witness high levels of distress, suffering, or trauma, researchers Singer and Klimecki argue that "empathic distress fatigue" is a better descriptor of this condition.[15] In a review on this topic in the *Canadian Veterinary Journal*, Tricia Dowling explains that, "compassion fatigue is a misnomer . . . it is empathy that fatigues in caregivers, not compassion." She adds, "Compassion does not fatigue—it is neurologically rejuvenating!"[16] Mindfulness appears to be a key component of compassion that protects from empathic distress fatigue. Mindful awareness (of our feelings, thoughts, beliefs, perceptions, and body responses) helps to avoid the trap of merging with another's pain, and instead fosters resilience, connection, caring, and resourceful action.[17]

Renowned vegan author and activist Colleen Patrick-Goudreau concurs: "I don't believe it is *compassion* that fatigues us, and I don't believe that we could ever have so much compassion that it would result in exhaustion, but I do believe that we can experience *empathic overarousal* or *empathic distress*, terms that are increasingly used by those who study burnout and that I think more accurately characterize exactly what is taking place. Empathy is important for understanding others' emotions, but feeling empathy can also be painful." She elaborates: "In other words, *empathic distress is the problem. Compassion is the remedy*."[18]

We will discuss empathic distress, and coping strategies to manage it, in more depth in Chapter Ten ("Thriving Emotionally and Socially as a Vegan").

Benefits of compassion

There are countless benefits to cultivating compassion. It is good not only for those we want to help; it is beneficial for us as well. Research shows that being compassionate is linked to positive psychological outcomes, including increased happiness, decreased depression and anxiety, decreased reactivity to stress, improved mental health, and better relationships. Compassion skills are fundamental to healthy connections with others, whether with our family, friends, colleagues, students, or patients.[19] Research suggests that while some of us may be more naturally compassionate, compassion can be learned. Those trained in compassion skills show increased prosocial behavior, along with reporting greater positive affect and resilience.[20]

In addition to personal benefits of compassion, there are many clear societal benefits. Compassion for those who suffer injustice has sparked many social justice movements and positive societal changes throughout history. Leaders of such movements, including Mahatma Gandhi, Martin Luther King Jr., Desmond Tutu, and Nelson Mandela, were known for their compassionate leadership. Compassionate role models, teachers, and leaders are key to creating a more peaceful and cooperative society that cares for the well-being of all. Importantly, compassion and prosocial behaviors are contagious. As each of us lives more compassionately, it sparks compassion in others.

What about compassion for animals?

While much of the discussion on compassion has centered around human-to-human relationships, it turns out that our treatment of animals and our compassion for them are important barometers of our mental health, as well as how we treat other humans. There is recognition in the mental health field that animal cruelty is a predictor of violence against humans,[21] while compassion and tenderness toward animals is associated with healthy prosocial behaviors.[22]

Additionally, connections with animals are healthy for us personally. You may have heard that bonding with animals improves our physical and mental health. Research shows that interacting with animals has been shown to lower blood pressure and decrease stress hormones such as cortisol. Our bonds with animals help us to feel less lonely and increase our emotional well-being. These bonds also strengthen children's social and emotional skills.[23]

What blocks our compassion?

We are taught from a young age that compassion toward others, including animals, is good. But most of us also learn, from the modeling of adults in our lives, to limit our compassion to select groups or species. It's natural for children to be curious about animals and to enjoy spending time with them. Many children adore companion animals, like to watch animals in nature, and enjoy going to petting zoos. However, there is an underlying message, often unspoken, that some animals are worthy of our caring and compassion, while others are not.

As children, we are encouraged in our love for certain animals, while at the same time being served meals centered around the flesh, secretions, and body parts of other animals. Because the cooked meat on our plate doesn't necessarily resemble the animal that it came from, we may not realize that what we are eating is an animal. If we do make the connection and ask questions, our parents or other authorities in our lives are likely to respond by justifying the practice of eating animals; for example, saying that we need meat and dairy to be healthy, or that certain animals are meant for food.

In our adulthood, we still might not make the connection between animal suffering and meat. The animal agriculture industry and other societal forces do all they can to hide and to justify the treatment of farmed animals. In addition, our social conditioning (i.e., the ingrained message that eating meat is natural, healthy, and even imperative) can block us from seeking to learn about animal agriculture and from making more informed and compassionate choices in what we buy and eat.

We may block our compassion to avoid the discomfort that comes with seeing what farmed animals go through. If we don't know, we don't have to feel. And it is true: watching the footage from factory farms and slaughterhouses can be greatly disturbing. When we witness and empathize with another's suffering, our own pain processing centers are activated. If we don't know how to cope with these feelings, it can lead to a sense of overwhelm and a desire to do whatever we can to avoid these intense emotions.

In addition, we may not want to know because we do not feel ready to change our behaviors around what we eat. We may believe that if we aren't willing or able to make big changes right away, why bother to learn more or make any changes at all? We may believe that our individual actions won't make a difference. We may fear that looking more closely at the treatment of animals in animal agriculture will move us out of our comfort zone—something many of us avoid.

Shifting your mindset to awaken compassion

How do we break through these barriers to expand our compassion for all sentient beings? How do we realize and experience the benefits of compassion for ourselves, for others, and for a world where all can flourish? My research participants and many other vegans have found that, even though acknowledging and empathizing with the suffering of animals can bring up tough emotions, the benefits of making compassionate choices far outweigh those of staying in the dark. The following are five suggestions for shifting your mindset to cultivate compassion.

1. **Recognize the personal benefits of extending compassion**. You may have fears that if you connect with animal suffering, you will get stuck in painful feelings and be overwhelmed (i.e., experience empathic distress). However, there are healthy ways to hold compassion that can lead to greater peace, well-being, and positive feelings. We will discuss coping strategies in Chapter Ten ("Thriving Emotionally and Socially as a Vegan"), but for now, I invite you to remember: The antidote to empathic distress is to move toward aligned, mindful, compassionate action. Our compassion guides us to bear witness and, when possible, do what we can to help others. Taking steps to lessen the suffering of others brings us greater peace and fulfillment. *You are not called to do it all, or to fix everything. Just allow your compassion to lead you to the next step that you feel called to take.*

2. **Get to know farm animals.** One of the best ways to do this is to visit a farm animal sanctuary. This gives us the opportunity to meet farmed animals close-up and see them as the unique individuals

that they are. There is nothing that breaks through our blocks to compassion more than developing a face-to-face connection. We discover firsthand that these sentient beings have personalities, intelligence, feelings, social relationships, and preferences, just as our companion animals do. Farm Sanctuary in Watkins Glen, New York,[24] has played a big role in awakening and nurturing my compassion for animals in the food system. I first visited early on my veg journey and have been a regular visitor ever since. Farm Sanctuary provides tours where you meet and interact with rescued animals, including cows, sheep, goats, chickens, and turkeys. Through these tours, I have been touched by each animal's individuality and their playful and social natures. Since Farm Sanctuary's start in 1986, many other farm animal sanctuaries have been established across the United States and globally.

3. **Witness the realities of modern animal agriculture.** Many of us have images of bucolic farm scenes, with cows or sheep frolicking in the countryside, until we dare to take a deeper look. Often, watching a video that shows what happens in factory farms and slaughterhouses is the turning point to awakening compassion. Before seeing it, we are disconnected. Once we see it, we can't unsee it. Consider checking out a video like *Meet Your Meat* or *Dairy Is Scary*,[25] which share the actualities of factory farming in about five to ten minutes. For a more in-depth understanding, watch some documentaries, perhaps starting with *Vegucated*, *The Peaceable Kingdom*, or *Cowspiracy*.[26] If you are ready to go further in facing truths about animal exploitation, check out *Earthlings* or *Dominion*.[27] These last two are not easy to watch, but both are credited with opening the eyes and hearts of countless people. I watched *Earthlings* when considering going vegan, and it was the impetus that launched me into a fully vegan lifestyle. It connected me with my grief and sadness about animal suffering in a way that nothing else had. Although it was difficult and painful, afterward I felt cleansed, as I acknowledged fully what I had subconsciously known but tried to avoid. Knowing I could make the decision to stop contributing to this suffering gave me a sense of freedom and empowerment.

4. **Find positive vegan role models** who show that veganism is not only possible and sustainable, but also transformational. If you don't know any vegans in your immediate network, join vegan or plant-based groups locally or online. Once you have vegan support and learn how to *thrive* with a plant-based lifestyle, it is easier to open your compassion for the sentient beings in the animal agriculture system. Find vegan groups that embody values that matter to you, whether you want to help animals, improve your health, heal from disease, and/or heal the planet. As you learn from role models and teachers who embody the positives of this lifestyle, you'll be on the path toward your own compassionate journey.

5. **Don't forget self-compassion**. We each have our own process of change and our unique feelings and experiences along the way. Hold compassion for the ups and downs you may experience as you make changes, and for the feelings that are triggered. Include yourself in your circle of compassion and prioritize healthy self-care, such as stress management skills, mindfulness practices, compassionate self-talk, adequate sleep and renewal, and high-nutrient plant foods. In Chapter Ten, I will discuss the benefits of self-compassion and self-care in more depth.

"Radical compassion is rooted in mindful, embodied presence, and it is expressed actively through caring that includes all beings."
—**Tara Brach**, Ph.D., in *Radical Compassion*[28]

Compassion is worth it

The majority of my research participants expressed that, despite the discomfort and challenges of awakening compassion, it was well worth it. One participant noted: "My sense of compassion for all living things is enhanced. It feels good to make a commitment and stick to it, even when it isn't convenient." Another indicated that she tries to focus on the ways she can have an impact: "I feel much more connected with my compassion and empathy. I focus on things I can control, and I try to be the change I want to see in the world."

What follows are the stories of two women who embody the healing power of compassion. In my interviews with them, Anita and Nancy each shared their awakening to compassion for all sentient beings, and how this expanded compassion has touched their lives and guided their actions.

Anita's story

Anita is a retired nurse and a graduate of Main Street Vegan Academy (MSVA).[29] She noted a love of animals and nature going back to childhood. She was inspired to go vegan to improve her health after attending her first Veg Fest in 2010. She was vegan for a year and a half, but then went back to eating local eggs, dairy, and "wild" salmon. However, after a health scare with ductal carcinoma in situ (stage zero breast cancer), she began to revisit the idea of a vegan lifestyle. "I thought, what is the healthiest diet? In the back of my mind, I knew that a fully plant-based diet was healthiest." She returned to Veg Fest in 2019, and "it was just the right moment." She explained:

> Recently, I had spent time with a friend who was vegan, and she said something very heartfelt about the plight of food animals that moved me. I was touched but also perplexed. I wondered, "What should I make of it? Why does she feel this? What allows her to feel, when I don't?"
>
> That planted a seed. When I went to Veg Fest this time, I was finally open and ready to hear the message. There was a big difference when I connected with the spiritual component of being vegan. The health message is one thing that impacted me, but that can be distorted because there's so much confusing information out there. The spiritual message spoke to my heart. And when I looked at the planet and the animals and brought it all together, I got it. It penetrated a different part of me. It wasn't just my head. It was that heart and gut connection.
>
> It hit something so deep inside of me, and it was a transformation that I can't undo. I'm a changed person because of this and I can't undo that . . . even though there was pain because my heart was more open. Connecting with animals' suffering and my own suffering was painful and brought up grief.

I'm not a person who likes to express anger. But I could sometimes feel this rage about the suffering of animals and others not getting it. I mean, how can we possibly have all these degrees of separation between ourselves and animals in order to continue to eat them? I think once you've removed some of those layers, it's like an onion—there's always the potential to peel off another . . . there's that potential for opening up even more.

In the past, my focus for social justice stuff was always about humans, but there is something about connecting with animals that is so pure. They don't have all the accumulated armor that we humans have, and they just are who they are. There's something about seeing and connecting with them that is so powerful.

Being vegan has enhanced my connection to the natural world and ability to take solace in it. Like for instance, watching my dog die. She was so stoic. Now I really look out at the trees and watch the squirrels. It's like I'm more connected with this cycle of life and death and not apart from it. To me, there's deep solace in that.

As a spiritual person, I believe that we are here to do our best and contribute something positive in any way we can. I think a vegan world means a compassionate world. I do believe that killing animals is really at the root of all violence. I realize that's an awfully strong statement. But that shift in consciousness could shift everything. There are days that I feel down, but I realize whatever negativity I have, what good does that do? What does that help? I need to have compassion for myself when I feel that way because I think it's very understandable . . . but it's not a mindset to stay in.

I'm so grateful my path led me here. I wish it had happened earlier, but I was definitely working my way toward it for a long time—becoming vegan and all the growth that goes with that. I feel like it's connected me back to myself. It's made me more of who I am and who I was. It has connected me to my essential self. I'm less focused on the outer self, more in touch with who I truly am and what is important to me.

Nancy P.'s story

Nancy Poznak is the founder of BotaniCuisine and owner of Wild Heart Bistro in Baltimore, Maryland.[30] She became vegetarian at age 16 as part of a spiritual quest. "I learned that all nutrition starts in plants." In her twenties, she lapsed back into eating animal products, but years later, came across some videos about animal agriculture. She stated, "I was devastated. Determined to learn the truth, I dove into researching the many aspects of using animals for food and other purposes. What I discovered made it evident I had to go vegan." Fairly quickly, she began to experience a profound sense of appreciation for the lives and sentience of non-human animals. She described an expanded awareness that brought greater empathy and compassion for all beings, along with great joy. She said:

> I came to realize that it's unethical to turn sentient beings of any species into commodities. Regardless of "humane" treatment, using others for what their bodies produce is always exploitative and harmful.
>
> This has brought me to a great awakening. I used to think animals were two-dimensional. When we primarily perceive others in terms of their utility, we don't fully see them. We disregard their capacities for sentience, love, and social connection. Our use of animals is especially horrible because it's not necessary. This is why I do the work I do—creating vegan food. The perceived utility of using and eating animals is a primary barrier for embracing veganism. Before people can embrace animal rights, they need to know that there is a way to live without eating animals.
>
> I have found a great sense of purpose and joy in being a vegan advocate. I no longer have to shut down a part of myself to engage in eating or using animals, which has helped my emotional and psychological well-being.
>
> My actions are part of the solution to end the immense suffering and destruction caused by animal industries. My purpose is to contribute to the greater good. Being vegan springs from my heart. I've come to realize that living vegan is aligned with our shared values of kindness, compassion, and caring about the earth and all those with whom we share our planet. As human beings, we are meant to experience love and peace and to express kindness to others, and to think of others, not just ourselves.

Anita's and Nancy's stories share how awakening their compassion for all sentient beings has deepened their own lives and led to greater fulfillment and authenticity. As we have discovered, there are many societal and financial forces that try to distance us from even knowing about the conditions in which farmed animals live and die. And our own inner blocks further distance us from making these connections and expanding our compassion. Yet, the research on compassion, and the experience of many vegans, shows that broadening our circle of compassion can be an experience that ultimately frees us as well as others around us.

Awakening my natural compassion was one of the greatest gifts that being vegan has given me. Extending compassion to others, especially the vulnerable and the voiceless, brings more meaning and fullness to our human experience and moves us toward creating a kinder, healthier, and more sustainable world where all can flourish.

Action Steps

The following are reflections and activities to support you in awakening and cultivating your compassion.

- **Set an intention.** Write in your journal: In what ways do you wish to cultivate your compassion? For example:
  - o Extend greater compassion toward those different than you.
  - o Develop more understanding and empathy for those with whom you disagree.
  - o Be proactive in learning about injustices for animals, workers, and others in the production of your food and other purchases.
  - o Show greater compassion and kindness toward yourself.
- **Reflection question:** Think about experiences you have had with animals throughout your life, including your pets, visits to zoos, times in nature, or seeing farm animals. Write in your journal, using these questions as prompts:
  - o How have these animals touched your life?
  - o What have you learned from them?
  - o What has moved you or intrigued you in these experiences?
  - o What has been painful or difficult?
  - o What has been healing or heartwarming?
- **Reflection question:** Journal about what compassion means to you, drawing on the following prompts:
  - o How have you expressed compassion in your life?
  - o What has been positive about these experiences, and what has been difficult?

o If your experience of compassion has been painful or difficult in some way, reflect on why. What has contributed to this?

o Do you need to release misconceptions or myths about compassion? For example:

- The myth that compassion means being soft and sentimental. If you don't identify as "warm and fuzzy" or as an "animal lover," realize that neither of these are prerequisites for choosing a cruelty-free lifestyle. Consider this: It takes courage and tenacity to go against the status quo and take a stand that all beings deserve a life that is free from unnecessary suffering.

- The myth that compassion means being a martyr or that you are personally responsible for ending all suffering. Healthy compassion includes recognizing that you, too, are a sentient being, and acknowledging your own feelings, needs, and limits. If you are a highly empathic person and struggle with this, please check out the suggestions in Chapter Ten and the Resources section at the back of the book.

- **Watch a documentary** about animal agriculture and its impact on animals, the environment, and/or human health. In addition to the videos and documentaries listed earlier in this chapter, there is a list of documentaries in the Resources section at the back of this book.

- **Plan a trip to a farm sanctuary.** Check online to find an animal sanctuary near you.[31]

- **Practice loving-kindness meditation.** The loving-kindness meditation (also called metta meditation) helps to connect with compassion for yourself, others, and all sentient beings. Regular practice has been associated with improved emotional regulation, decreased distress, greater resilience, improved relationships, and increased compassion.[32] There are many variations of this meditation available online. The following are basic instructions that I have used for my own practice and with clients. If you'd like, you can listen to a recording of this meditation on my website.[33]

  o ***Start with sending loving-kindness toward yourself.*** You need to fill your cup first before it can overflow to others. This is especially important if you tend to strongly identify with others' suffering. Close your eyes, if that feels comfortable, or hold a soft gaze. Say the following phrases silently: *May I be peaceful. May I be happy. May I be free from suffering.* (You can add other phrases as desired. For example: *May I be filled with loving-kindness. May I be healthy. May I be safe.*) Just breathe in these words. Repeat the phrases two or three times. Sometimes it helps to envision yourself as a child and send these loving-kindness wishes to your younger self as well.

o **Next, think of someone you love**. Picture their face and send the loving-kindness wishes to them: *May you be peaceful. May you be happy. May you be free from suffering.* You can add other phrases as you like: *May you be safe. May you be healthy and well.*

o **Extend the loving-kindness wishes to others you love**: *May you be peaceful. May you be happy. May you be free from suffering.*

o **Think of those you are concerned about**, those going through a hard time (whether you know them personally or not). Send the loving-kindness wishes to them. *May you be peaceful. May you be happy. May you be free from suffering.*

o **To deepen your practice,** send loving-kindness toward someone with whom you have a difficult relationship or whom you dislike: *Just as I want to be peaceful, may you be peaceful. Just as I want to be at ease, may you be at ease. Just as I want to be free from suffering, may you be free from suffering.*

o **Last of all, extend loving-kindness to all beings**. Picture the whole of nature and all sentient beings: *May all beings everywhere be peaceful, happy, and free.*

o **Bring closure to your practice.** Take a few deep breaths, open your eyes, and hold the intention to bring this loving-kindness into your actions today.

Living congruently with our values and awakening our compassion lays the foundation for more authentically sharing who we are in our connections with others. Aligning with our compassionate nature gives a greater sense of meaning to our lives. The next chapter explores the crucial importance that meaning and purpose play in a fulfilling life, and how for many vegans, a plant-powered, cruelty-free, and sustainable lifestyle becomes a key part of how they serve their purpose in the world.

CHAPTER 4

CONNECT WITH DEEPER MEANING AND PURPOSE

"Self-actualizing people are, without one single exception, involved in a cause outside their own skin, in something outside of themselves."

—Abraham Maslow

"The purpose of human life is to serve, and to show compassion and the will to help others."

—Albert Schweitzer

Finding my voice through veganism

I've always sought a sense of meaning and purpose in my life. This search for meaning ultimately led to my career in psychology. Through continuing education and my work with psychotherapy clients, I was able to study, learn, teach, connect, and impact others in ways that resonated with my gifts and passions. As I supported clients on their journeys to heal from trauma, cope with the stresses and losses of life, become healthier, and develop healthier relationships with themselves and others, I found deep fulfillment. I was guided by a holistic view of well-being, empowering my clients (and myself) to thrive in mind, body, and spirit.

Over time, I became more attuned to the social and systemic issues that impact our well-being, problems like inequity, poverty, racism, sexism, violence, and other injustices. I longed for a world that was kinder and more just for all. My vegan journey further increased my recognition of the ways that entrenched societal systems and structures often contribute to harm and oppression of those with less power, including those with lower socioeconomic status, immigrants, minorities, and non-human animals who are exploited and commodified.

I came to realize that being vegan brings together many of the issues that really matter to me. Veganism is a way of living that minimizes harm and exploitation of sentient beings, to the best of our ability. I found that by not buying, eating, or consuming products sourced from animals, I can make a difference for many problems I deeply care about: animal rights and well-being, the flourishing of our planet, and human health. Through this choice, I can contribute toward a more sustainable way of living, for my own health and longevity, for others, for the environment, and for food availability for all. In addition, I realized that bringing greater compassion to all sentient beings is a critical step in healing the disconnection and violence that pervades our world. I saw that vegan issues, such as how we treat animals and the food choices we make, affect our mental health and emotional well-being. There are many world events that cause me great distress that I can do very little about. However, each day I have a choice of what I eat and purchase, and these choices can have a huge impact.

Upon making these powerful connections, veganism became more than a personal dietary choice for me. It strengthened the sense of purpose I already found through my work and became a passion that focused my daily activities and life direction. It became a calling to model, inspire, and teach so that I could help others and move the societal needle toward vegan values. Subsequently, I've been on a quest to discover how I can use my gifts, skills, and experience to share the benefits and vital importance of this lifestyle with others. Despite my natural tendency to be quiet and private, my passion about these issues has led me to speak out in ways that I hadn't anticipated, from writing a blog, to speaking and teaching, to writing this book. Through it all, there is a deep sense of purpose, an inner drive to play my part in contributing to a kinder, healthier, and more sustainable world.

Our search for meaning and purpose

Philosophers, psychologists, inspirational speakers, and theologians all agree that meaning and purpose are central to a life well lived. Victor Frankl, psychiatrist, Holocaust survivor, and author of *Man's Search for*

Meaning, argued that the quest for meaning is one of the primary tasks of our existence.[1] Meaning is involved in how we make sense of our life and our experiences. Our life feels meaningful when we experience it as having significance, value, coherence, and purpose.[2] *Purpose* refers to our direction in life, having intentions and goals that motivate us. Our purpose inspires us toward actions that are personally meaningful *and* create positive change in the world.[3]

Having a greater sense of meaning and purpose is associated with improved life satisfaction, increased happiness, and decreased depression,[4] as well as greater physical well-being, cognitive functioning, and longevity.[5] Our sense of meaning and purpose adds richness to life and brings a sense of coherence and guidance even through loss and difficulties.

During Victor Frankl's imprisonment in Nazi concentration camps, in which millions of prisoners died, he found that fellow prisoners who sustained a sense of purpose were more likely to survive. Dr. Frankl himself found deep meaning in the hope of reuniting with loved ones, as well as holding a vision of sharing his learnings with the world. His discoveries and experiences ultimately shaped his professional contribution after he was freed at the end of World War II. His teachings and insights around the centrality of meaning, and our ability to choose how we respond to our circumstances, continue to greatly influence modern existential and humanistic psychology principles.[6]

Our sense of purpose appears to be integral to our health and longevity, as shown by those living in the Blue Zones, geographic regions with higher-than-average numbers of individuals living long, healthy, and active lives even into their hundreds. Dan Buettner, best-selling author and National Geographic Fellow, has visited and researched these areas for decades. He notes that along with a plant-strong diet, daily movement, and strong social connections, a sense of purpose is an intrinsic facet of life for Blue Zone residents. He speaks of the Japanese concept of *ikigai*, which is translated as "Why I wake up in the morning." Residents of the Blue Zones express a sense that they have something to contribute, a reason for waking with joy each day. This in turn contributes to staying involved in their communities, daily tasks, and meaningful activities.[7]

Nuances of purposeful living

While having a sense of meaning and purpose contributes to greater overall happiness and fulfillment, a meaningful life does not mean that we are happy all the time. As we make sense of the tragedies in our lives and in the world around us, we will likely struggle with difficult emotions. And as we become more aware of the animal suffering, environmental degradation, and harm to humans that result from factory farming and other exploitative industries, it is normal to feel sadness or anger. A meaningful life is one in which we incorporate our whole self and all our experiences into a coherent whole. We may not always have answers, but we try to make sense of what is happening and take the best steps we know to take in an imperfect world. We are no longer "blissfully" ignorant, but instead experience the full tapestry of emotions that are part of being an aware, compassionate human being.

Although living a meaningful life does not guarantee an individual's happiness, meaningfulness and happiness are highly correlated. That is, those who experience more meaning tend to be happier (and vice versa). Feeling connected to others, having a sense of belonging, and feeling productive are common factors that contribute to both happiness and a sense of meaning. However, there are some important differences between these two states as well. *Happiness* is commonly defined as a sense of subjective well-being, life satisfaction, and/or positive mood, while *meaning* relates to whether we assess our lives as having value and purpose.

A study by Roy Baumeister and colleagues explored "key differences between a happy life and a meaningful life."[8] The researchers found that happiness tended to be present-focused, and was associated with satisfying one's wants and needs, feeling good emotionally, and having fewer life struggles. In contrast, meaningfulness integrated the past, present, and future. Meaning was uniquely associated with doing positive things for others, being more of a giver, and taking part in activities that expressed and reflected one's identity and values. Interestingly, having a higher sense of meaning was also associated with higher stress, anxiety, worry, and even arguments. The authors theorized that when we are engaged in meaningful activities, things that really matter to us and make a difference, we may experience greater stress and worry, as well as disagreements over these issues. The authors state, "We propose that meaningfulness comes in part from being involved in things one regards as important, and sometimes one has to argue for these."[9]

Challenges, stress, and struggles are inextricably interwoven with our search for greater meaning. And at the same time, as we cultivate meaning through our life experiences, this often leads to greater fulfillment, happiness, and finding our authentic purpose. In the process of making sense of the events in our own lives and in the world around us, we are often guided to contribute our unique gifts to create positive change in the world. As explained in the book *True Purpose*, we yearn to know why we are here and what we are meant to contribute. The author, Tim Kelley, elaborates, "Sustained happiness comes from meaning. It comes from growing, developing, and having a positive impact on the lives of others."[10]

Often the problems or situations that cause us the greatest distress are ones that we ultimately feel called to change or heal—within ourselves, as well as in the world. As you will read, this is the experience of many vegans who, upon learning about the harmful impact of animal agriculture on animal well-being, human health, social justice, and the planet, feel called to shift their own behaviors, and ultimately to raise awareness and bring about larger societal change.

Veganism and purpose

When asked about ways that being vegan contributed to their emotional well-being, three-quarters of my survey respondents reported a greater sense of meaning and purpose associated with becoming vegan. This sense of meaning infiltrated numerous aspects of their lives, ranging from the personal fulfillment of living aligned with values of compassion, health, and sustainability, to engaging in volunteer activities or work that helped to promote these values.

Many vegan participants expressed a deep sense of purpose simply through choosing not to purchase food or other items created through the harm, suffering, or exploitation of animals, as shown in the sampling of survey responses here:

"I feel a greater sense of purpose in knowing that I am doing what I can to not bring more harm and trauma to the earth and the creatures with whom we share it."

"Knowing that I am doing what I can to reduce suffering gives my life meaning."

"I now live with purpose, a sense of contributing to the greater good, and making mindful choices."

"Knowing that I'm making choices that support compassion-based foods and products, knowing that my purchase decisions contribute even a little to the end of animal suffering, grounds me in love and gratitude."

"I know I am on the right path now, being vegan. I have always wanted to be an ethical person who is in tune with deeper meaning in life. Veganism is how I achieve a deep, ethical life, expanding my concern for others and myself on so many levels . . . I feel like I'm doing what I came here to do in the larger scheme of life, that I'm finally living a life of meaning, contributing to something greater than myself."

In addition, many of my study participants reported a sense of purpose through actively working to share the benefits of veganism with others and to create positive change in the world. They did this through a range of activities, such as sharing on social media, bringing enticing vegan food to social events, gardening, writing blogs, creating podcasts, and advocating for veganism in their work and/or personal lives. Some wrote books on vegan issues. Numerous others worked for, or volunteered with, vegan organizations. And many created vegan businesses, including restaurants, catering, cooking classes, nutritional and health coaching, fitness guidance, consulting, training, and producing a variety of plant-based and vegan products.

Next I share some of the diverse ways that my research interviewees contribute their gifts and serve their purpose.

Advocating for animals

The majority of my vegan participants (81 percent) reported that compassion for animals was a primary factor in their decision to become vegan. An even greater number (92 percent said that it played a huge role in convincing them to *stay* vegan.[11] Upon learning about the suffering of animals in agriculture and other industries, many respondents felt called to advocate on behalf of animals. They did this through writing books, articles, or social media posts; creating educational programs to raise awareness; engaging in protests or vigils; and working for animal sanctuaries or animal protection organizations.

One of my interviewees, Cheryl Moss, became an author to raise awareness and awaken compassion for farmed animals. She said, "Fighting for animals has become my life's purpose. I have written three children's books on this subject, created a website, and am building my final chapter with passion for this cause." Her website, *Better Life For Animals*, shares wisdom and resources for how kids and their parents can make changes that help farm animals.

Michelle Schaefer (whose story is shared in Chapter Eight) stated, "I've learned that action is the antidote to depression, helplessness, and even anger. For a long time, I was 'just' a vegan. Now I'm a vegan activist. Veganism is my everything. I started a vegan meetup in my community, penned a Meatless Monday article in my local paper, and later became a vegan staff writer for a magazine."

Another interviewee, Jane Velez-Mitchell, brought her expertise as an award-winning television news reporter and anchor to create UnchainedTV, a free global streaming television network that focuses on the plant-based lifestyle and related issues, such as animal protection, health, and the environment. This network streams documentaries, news, cooking shows, talk shows, biographies, and music, all aimed to support people toward greater awareness of the benefits of plant-based living for animals, humans, and the planet. Jane passionately speaks about these issues through her reporting and expert interviews on her podcast (available on UnchainedTV).

Sharing tantalizing and nourishing vegan food

Several participants found their purpose through sharing the deliciousness of vegan food, in their personal lives and/or professionally. I was surprised to discover the variety of ways that this was expressed: being a vegan chef, caterer, or cooking instructor; opening a vegan restaurant or food stall; creating cookbooks or food blogs; consulting with and training local restaurants; and creating commercial foods or supplements.

Sharing wholesome and delectable vegan food is foundational to opening minds to the possibilities of plant-powered living. Until we taste how delicious it can be, we may not see how this way of living can be possible or desirable. Thus, creating nourishing food for others can be a powerful form of activism. As expressed by a vegan restaurant owner: "We are the change and through my food, I can reach so many people. I feel that I can make a small change to a huge problem, but collectively, we can have a massive impact." Another survey respondent said, "I have started a vegan bakery business as well as a vegan food blog, both of which feel so aligned with my purpose and bring me so much joy."

One interviewee, Meredith Marin, brought her education and experience to create a business as a vegan hospitality consultant. When she became vegan, she found that not many vegan options were available in local eateries and saw the need to help restaurants attune to vegan and plant-based consumers. Subsequently, she worked with restaurants, hotels, chefs, and food service businesses to train staff to provide enticing vegan options. Following her extensive work with restaurants and chefs in Aruba, it became recognized as the most vegan-friendly island in the Caribbean due to its tantalizing vegan culinary scene. She has since created a Vegan Hospitality Consultant Certification program to train other vegans to offer similar consultancy services in their own communities. Meredith said, "Being vegan changed my whole life. It added to my sense of purpose in life, in parenting, and in my career."

Many expressed fulfillment and purpose through bringing enticing vegan meals to family and social events. As shared by one participant: "It was becoming vegan that elevated my cooking from really good home cooking to restaurant-worthy and magazine-worthy artistic creations. I love to give people exquisitely scrumptious vegan food, and have them walk away from the table saying, 'That might have been the best meal I've ever had in my damn life.' I feel a sense of purpose in being able to do that."

Modeling the health and fitness benefits

Vegans who personally discover the healing power of a plant-based lifestyle often feel called to bring their experience to help others gain better health. My research respondents included physicians and other healthcare professionals who had redirected their professional practices to support patients in adopting a plant-based diet and healthy lifestyle practices. Other participants were plant-based health, nutrition, or fitness coaches. Some created or worked for organizations that raise awareness of the benefits of plant-based nutrition for one's health. Some wrote books or articles about their own healing and/or the scientific evidence supporting a plant-based diet. Others were vegan athletes or bodybuilders.

One respondent, Dr. Akil Taher, a physician, author, and motivational speaker, discovered a renewed sense of purpose after experiencing a personal health crisis. This pivotal moment led him to adopt a whole-food, plant-based diet. Driven by his transformative journey, he now dedicates himself to raising awareness and guiding others toward healthy lifestyle changes. He shared his inspiring story in his book, *Open Heart*, which chronicles his journey from undergoing bypass surgery at age 61 to running marathons and mountain climbing. His example highlights the profound impact of a plant-based diet, mental and emotional resilience, and spiritual growth in finding life's purpose. He now dedicates most of his time to giving educational talks that focus on preventing and treating the cause of chronic diseases, rather than treating the consequence of disease after the fact.

Geoff Palmer, vegan body-building champion and founder of a plant-based fitness supplement company, has found his purpose through educating others about the science of plant-based nutrition for health and fitness. He expressed a special passion for raising awareness among men. He said, "I have been vegan for thirty-eight years, eating nothing but plants. I read a stat that 80 percent of vegans in the United States are women; only 20 percent are men. That's a horrible disparity. The dogma and mindset that 'meat is masculinity' is pervasive. I really want to try to help break through that. I focus on the science and the physical fitness aspect to help create a shift so that men can better receive the message."

Raising awareness through plant-based businesses

Several research participants found purpose in bringing their business expertise to support plant-based, eco-oriented, and/or ethical businesses and organizations. Recognizing that plant-based products and services are crucial for creating a vegan world, these professionals offer services such as consulting, marketing, public relations, content creation, training, and coaching to help vegan entrepreneurs and companies thrive.

After becoming vegan, Kathleen Gage, a marketing consultant, podcaster, and author, brought her nearly three decades of experience to found Vegan Visibility, a business that supports vegan and plant-based entrepreneurs and authors in sharing their message and mission. During our interview, she said, "Like many people, when I went plant-based, I realized, this is the holy grail of living and eating. I got my plant-based nutrition certificate from eCornell University and thought I was going to be a nutrition coach. I then realized that I have very little patience for that. That is not my wheelhouse at all." Kathleen ultimately realized that her purpose would be better served through drawing on her passions, skills, and extensive experience to empower vegan business owners and leaders to have a bigger impact.

Sandra Nomoto, who provides marketing, coaching, consulting, and other services for vegan businesses and authors, shared how becoming vegan contributed to her greater purpose. She said, "Being vegan has been the missing puzzle piece in my life without me realizing it. Since I was young, I've wanted to live in a socially and environmentally conscious way and I knew subconsciously that eating vegan was one way to do it. It wasn't until I transitioned to a vegan diet in 2018 that I felt I was really living according to the values I preached. In 2019, I received intuitive guidance with regards to my career, which is related to veganism. Now I feel like both my work and personal life as a vegan contribute to my purpose." Sandra subsequently authored the book, *Vegan Marketing Success Stories*.

Andrea Learned used her extensive background in marketing and communications to empower sustainability-oriented leaders and influencers, and to help their message reach more people. She said, "My [plant-based] adventure was first for health reasons, then the climate, and then later an awareness of the animal impact. Now I'm a strategic advisor for businesses to make their climate leadership more visible. I view both personal diet choice and organizational food policy as incredibly powerful but as-yet untapped climate influence levers." Andrea hosts a podcast, *Living Change: A Quest for Climate Leadership*.

Creating vegan communities

Several study participants found purpose through leading local plant-based groups and communities, aiming to raise awareness and provide support for people interested in adopting a plant-based or vegan lifestyle. These groups provide restaurant meet-ups, potlucks, expert presentations, education, and cooking demos. Since the pandemic, some groups have developed a following beyond their local communities through online events.

Sally Lipsky, founder of Plant-Based Pittsburgh, brought her expertise as a retired professor of education to teach others about the benefits of a plant-based lifestyle, after healing from cancer. She said, "I took my background in education and created a local plant-based community group. We have cooking demos, classes on meal prep, and educational programs that make plant-based eating more accessible." Sally's story is shared in more depth in Chapter Seven.

Leader of Plant Powered Metro New York (PPMNY), Lianna Levine Reisner, said, "My sense of purpose and my strong understanding of the many arguments for healthy vegan living keep me energized. I co-founded an organization to provide education and support to others on the path to a plant-based lifestyle, which has led to an influx of many volunteers, advisors, staff, and community members who are all committed to the same lifestyle and support each other in turn." PPMNY empowers diverse communities to overcome chronic disease and gain better health through educational programs about the power of whole-food, plant-based nutrition.

Some vegans express their purpose through raising awareness on a national or global scale. For example, Wanda Huberman is the executive director for the National Health Association (NHA), the longest-running nonprofit vegan organization in the United States. Founded in 1948, the NHA provides yearly conferences with plant-based experts, as well as an educational magazine, podcast, newsletter, and exciting vegan travel opportunities, all aimed to promote a whole-food, plant-based lifestyle for holistic health. Wanda started at her current position in 2020, after thirty years in another industry. During our interview, she enthusiastically shared how meaningful this work is for her personally, as she herself has experienced greatly improved health through a whole-plant-food diet. Further, it has created the opportunity to work alongside her husband, Mark Huberman, president of NHA, in their shared passion for empowering and educating others to thrive with a plant-powered lifestyle.

Another venture of shared passion for veganism was the creation of Vegan Street by interviewee John Beske and his wife, Marla. First launched in 1998, Vegan Street is an educational website and newsletter that offers articles, guides, recipes, and other resources on all aspects of vegan living. Over the years, through Vegan Street and other initiatives (e.g., local vegan festivals), John and Marla have provided support, education, and community for those living, or curious about, a vegan lifestyle. John expressed a deep sense of meaning from his work: "I have dedicated my life to building a healthier, more compassionate, and sustainable world. This sense of purpose keeps me going every day."

The Appendix shares additional examples of the diverse ways that vegans serve their purpose through teaching, modeling, and advocating a plant-powered, vegan lifestyle.

The path to vegan purpose

Trends on LinkedIn, perhaps the largest professional network on the internet, highlight the growing number of vegan businesses, organizations, and professionals who are expressing their purpose in the plant-based realm. At the time of writing this book, a search on LinkedIn found over 27,000 vegan businesses listed. In addition, LinkedIn hosts several groups of vegan and plant-based professionals, each with thousands of members.

Why does adopting a vegan lifestyle so often contribute to meaning and purpose? I believe it's because the philosophy and practice of vegan living has the potential to solve many of the most imminent crises that we face personally, societally, and globally. As stated by Phillip Wollen in his foreword to the book *Food Is Climate*: "Veganism is the 'Swiss Army knife' of the future. One instrument solves our ethical, economic, environmental, water, health, and sustainability problems—and ends Animal Cruelty forever."[12] This realization of the multi-faceted impact of our food choices awakens us to the possibility that we each can contribute to healing not only ourselves, but also our world.

This desire to bring healing to others or the world often starts with our own personal transformation, whether healing from chronic health conditions, overcoming unhealthy eating patterns, and/or awakening emotionally or spiritually. Many vegans find that the beauty and simplicity of plant-centered meals feels deeply right, like a truth that we've forgotten, a truth obscured by the advertising and agendas of food corporations, cultural habits, and our own unhealthy addictions. Eating from the bounty of the plant kingdom aligns with our underlying desire to live more naturally and healthily, in ways that nourish our bodies, minds, and spirits, and that are more in harmony with nature.

Whatever our initial reason for going vegan, when we break through the limits of our cultural conditioning to embrace plant-powered living, we often want to share this transformative experience with others. We have found a path that brings us health and vibrancy; healing of disease; enjoyment of nourishing food; compassionate, sustainable, and cruelty-free living; and the potential to heal many of the ills in our world. There are countless ways that we can bring our unique gifts, interests, passions, and voices to share the power of this life-changing lifestyle. No wonder many of us who become vegan want to share it with the world.

Making a commitment

Dedication and commitment are key to cultivating greater meaning and purpose. This is certainly true with a vegan lifestyle. For many of us, change is a gradual process, and we can benefit from *any* movement toward a more plant-based lifestyle—including improved health, less cruelty to animals, and decreased environmental impact. However, there is something about making a *commitment* to a lifestyle pattern that brings growth and meaning in a way that merely dabbling in a behavior does not.

When I first learned about the ethical, environmental, and health impacts of factory farming, I knew I wanted to stop eating meat. However, it took me about four months to stop entirely. I reached a point where I was eating solely vegetarian foods at home, but at social gatherings, I still sometimes ate small amounts of meat, mainly because I didn't want to stand out or "offend" certain people. And then, one of the books I was reading made me question why I wasn't honoring my values fully. What was holding me back from committing to what I believed? Something shifted, and I made the decision that animal flesh was no longer on the menu for me, no matter who was serving it. This led me to speak up and share socially that I was no longer eating any meat. My identity shifted along with it. I wasn't just eating more vegetables and less meat, I was now a *vegetarian*, aligned with ethics of compassion and decreasing animal suffering.

A similar process happened when becoming vegan. I strongly believed in the moral and ethical reasons for abstaining from all animal products, yet I found myself pulled into the old societal "trance" when I was at certain social gatherings, especially with foods where dairy or eggs were not clearly visible. As I described in Chapter Three, the documentary *Earthlings* fully awakened me from this hypnosis and led me to a wholehearted commitment. In deciding that I would no longer buy or consume any animal products, I became *vegan*. My lifestyle now feels more fully aligned with my values of compassion, nonviolence, health, and sustainability.

It was in making the commitment to a vegan lifestyle that I found a deeper sense of purpose. This would not have occurred with a half-hearted approach. There was something about standing for what I believed in, and speaking up even when it felt inconvenient or difficult, that led me to a sense of fulfillment, meaning, and purpose. This in turn moved me to draw on my gifts, skills, and life experience to teach and share vegan values of compassion, health, and sustainability.

I invite you to take a moment to reflect on your personal intentions. What has led you to read this book? What changes are you hoping to make? For example, do you want to shift toward a plant-based lifestyle to improve your health or fitness? Do you feel called to explore veganism for ethical or environmental reasons? Are you a vegetarian or vegan who wants to live in a more aligned way and/or make a greater contribution to your purpose? Whatever your personal goals or intentions, whatever your WHY, I invite you to consider: What is the commitment you want to make? You may or may not be ready to make a commitment just yet, but keep in mind that the most healing and empowering transformations occur when you determine your intentions and make a commitment that moves you toward them. (I will dive into this more deeply in Chapter Nine, when I cover "Keys to Successful Lifestyle Change").

The commitment to vegan values and lifestyle is foundational in creating a deep sense of purpose for many vegans. This is beautifully exemplified in the story of Jacque Salomon, whose journey to healing herself and her family led to a greater purpose and contribution than she ever could have imagined.

Jacque's story

Jacque Salomon is a trauma-informed health and wellness coach, national speaker (including Harvard Medical School), author, and founder and executive director of the Seeds to Inspire Foundation.[13] She is also founder and CEO of Angel in the Stone Transformational Coaching. Her journey to a vegan lifestyle was catalyzed by family health crises. She, her ex-husband, and her two teenage sons were dealing with obesity and multiple medical issues, and the only solutions offered were medications and invasive procedures. She was still reeling from the grief of losing a son at age eleven. "My eldest son passed away and earned his angel wings due to an adverse pharmaceutical reaction. So, relying on medications was not an option I wanted." She added:

> In 2016, I just dove in and said, "Okay, I have to learn how to heal holistically, for my kids." I started feeling that spiritual call. Everything inside of me as a mom came raging to the surface and I knew intuitively that there was something else. That's what led me to watch *Forks Over Knives*. That was when I shifted dimensions. I could no longer be the woman that I was before I watched that documentary. I looked at my kids and realized, "I am literally loving my children to death."
>
> And that led me to adopt a whole-food, plant-based, no-oil lifestyle to address our obesity and chronic diseases. This wasn't because of aesthetics; obesity was interfering and causing other chronic diseases and creating these other symptoms. There were just

more and more pills—I'm not joking, we had two-gallon sized Ziploc bags of prescriptions. I realized, I have to do better for my kids, and I have to show them a better way.

After I saw *Forks Over Knives*, it was really painful. How did I not know? How is this possible? It's so important to me, my identity as a mother. Subsequently, I enrolled in the Center for Nutrition Studies for a plant-based nutrition certificate. As I studied, the guilt set in, because I realized that I was on a slow suicide, and I was taking my children with me.

And I got angry, so angry. You know, that was a good thing, because it activated that mama bear in me, and I was like, okay, you did this to me, you fooled me. But you are not going to use my kids, monetize their health, and take away their ability to know what's right and wrong, to make decisions for their bodies. I have to become an elder so that I can guide them. It inspired me to be better and learn more so that I could be there for them.

What I found most empowering was discovering that our bodies are miraculous. I started realizing that what I was consuming was interfering with the natural homeostasis of my body and its ability to thrive. I realized, "Every time I eat this, every time I drink this, I'm challenging my body, and I'm giving her challenges that she doesn't need." And I think the anger came in because I didn't realize I was playing a game, and that the price was my health. I was consenting [to foods that were undermining my, and my children's, health], and I didn't know that. I don't want to do that anymore. I'm gonna give my body what she needs to thrive. And that was whole-plant nutrition. When you provide the right ecosystem inside your body, your body thanks you, and you start feeling better. You think more clearly, you can focus better, you're more compassionate. Your body responds to restoring homeostasis, which I translated to love. And when you embody that, you can navigate this world differently. It brought awareness that health autonomy is mine to have. That's my right.

When you truly start feeling great, you recognize when you eat something that's not helpful for you by how your body responds. And when you start feeling great, you start craving foods that actually make you feel good. All of a sudden, those foods that don't make you feel good are not as pleasurable and not as enticing anymore.

With a whole-food, plant-based diet, I was able to reverse my obesity. I was able to relinquish 164 pounds of excess weight, and heal my Type 2 diabetes, heart arrhythmia, hypertension, restless leg syndrome, chronic insomnia, and gastric reflux. I'm now free of pharmaceuticals and chronic disease. And within a year, the four of us [me, my ex-husband, and two sons] were down 300 pounds as a family.

Jacque shared that, over time, she became aware of the larger impacts of a vegan lifestyle, for the well-being of humanity, animals, and the planet. She came to realize that "veganism is a spiritual movement of anti-oppression, anti-harm, and consistent love and justice." She also realized that her deepest core values had always been aligned with veganism:

My whole life, I was always against oppression, I was always fighting for what was right. I was always fighting for our ability to love and be who we are, to live in compassion and joy. I think what is most painful, I now realize I was programmed to ignore the plight of certain animals. I could feel their plight—I'm a deeply empathic person, I could always feel it. I couldn't look, but I could put the food on the plate, and I could feed it to my children, because it was so processed, and so removed from what it originally looked and sounded like.

I realized that I never really liked to consume flesh. My sister reminded me, "You've always been that way. You never really liked meat anyway." I started going back to my Puerto Rican ancestry. And I started cooking the way my great-grandmother and my grandmother did, using mostly vegetables, rice, and beans.

Jacque shared how becoming a whole-food, plant-based vegan helped her to heal emotionally as well:

I have realized that being a brown woman, in this time and place, has conditioned me to lose my voice, to be small, to default to what was wrong with me—and to fear stepping into what was right with me. I feel that through being vegan and whole-food plant-based, and really restoring that homeostasis in my body, I was able to heal the trauma that was in my muscles and in my central nervous system. Before, I didn't have the space, time, energy to deal with it, because I was too overwhelmed and inundated with suffering to listen to those little inner voices that wanted to come to the surface.

I would say it was like a spring cleaning; I was able to purge all the trauma that I was ingesting. Unconsciously, I was able to forgive myself, which released a lot of space energetically in my body. And I was able to sit with all those traumas in my life. I was able to look at people and circumstances in my life through a lens of higher awareness and higher consciousness, and love my way through the pain, which I didn't have the capacity, the language, or the skills to do previously.

I'm a mom, first and foremost; it's the fire that fuels me. When my son passed away, that broke me open. That sent me on this journey to do what I do . . . to take my healing journey, and discover how to make this accessible to everyone. We're one family. The more we remember that, the more we're going to usher in the world that we deserve and that our babies deserve.

Jacque went on to create the Seeds to Inspire Foundation, which partners with other organizations to offer educational programs and mentoring in plant-based nutrition and healthy lifestyle, with a focus on marginalized and underserved communities that lack ready access to healthy foods. Her work has launched her into a leadership role in which she advocates for food justice, anti-oppression, and the well-being of humans, animals, and the environment.

When I met with Jacque for our interview, she spoke with such compassion, conviction, clarity, and passion it was clear that not only was her own life transformed by her plant-based healing, but that it was also a catalyst for larger-scale healing of the many people and communities whose lives she touches. Her work exemplifies how veganism connects many seemingly distinct issues, including personal health, public health, emotional healing, social justice, nurturing the earth, and anti-oppression for animals and humans.

As you reflect on the stories and examples in this chapter, how do they inspire your own sense of purpose? It's my personal belief that we each have a purpose, which is tied up in humanity's larger purpose. I believe that living our purpose, although it may bring challenges and pain at times, ultimately creates our greatest fulfillment. We each can make a difference through our choices. Our individual steps may feel small, but when we each contribute our part, we create momentum and synergy. As each of us shares our individual gifts, we are part of a greater whole, serving in ways that align with our unique nature, skills, passions, and calling. And when we each wholeheartedly offer our unique contribution, all of life can flourish.

Action Steps

The reflections and actions that follow are designed to help you gain more clarity about your purpose and identify your next steps for living with more meaning and purpose. Use your journal to write down your reflections and responses.

- **What issues, causes, or problems do you care most deeply about?** Consider the following reflections to help you gain clarity:
  - Imagine you are in conversation with someone. What conversation topic(s) would lead you to lean forward, talk faster, and become increasingly animated?
  - What topics or issues are you fascinated to read or learn more about?
  - If you had a magic wand and could fix one problem in the world, what would it be?
  - What problem or issue in our world makes you most angry?
  - Who or what are you helping when you feel most yourself and most fulfilled?
- **What do you love to do?**
  - What activities do you become so engrossed in that you lose track of time?
  - What activities or experiences energize you?
  - What do you love doing so much you'll do it even if you're not paid?
- **What are you really skilled at?**
  - What skills and abilities have you honed during your various work experiences?
  - What activities do you excel in?
  - What do other people tell you that you excel at?
  - What comes naturally to you that others seem to find more difficult?
- **What experiences have deeply impacted your life?** This can include positive experiences, as well as painful or difficult experiences or losses.

- **Examine your answers to the preceding questions, and reflect:**
  - o What do your responses show you about your purpose?
  - o In what ways are you already bringing your skills, passions, and experiences to help others and/or causes that matter to you?
  - o Does it feel like something is missing when it comes to serving your purpose?
  - o If YES, brainstorm possible ways to serve the causes that really matter to you.
  - o Pick one or two of the options that are most appealing and take action to implement or explore further. You may need to try out different options before you find something that really fits—something you love *and* that makes a positive impact. This may be a discovery process that evolves over time.
- **Wise Advisor meditation.** This exercise takes you beyond the limits of what you know with your rational brain, to connect with your inner guidance and wisdom. Sometimes we are restricted by what we "know" or have experienced in the past and get stuck in old ruts. This visualization helps to connect with greater creativity and possibility.[14] Keep an open mind and see what unfolds, following these instructions:[15]
  - o Find a comfortable place where you will not be disturbed. After getting comfortable, close your eyes or soften your gaze. Take five slow, deep breaths, and start to quiet your mind and body.
  - o Imagine yourself in a peaceful place. This can be a place in nature, or a favorite room or building. It can be somewhere you have been before, or a place you create in your own imagination. It could be by the ocean, in a forest, by a lake or stream, in a meadow, or in a calm and beautiful indoor space. Choose a setting that is peaceful or enjoyable for you. Picture it, drawing on all your senses: the sights, sounds, textures, feelings, and smells. Notice if you are sitting, standing, walking, or moving in some way.
  - o Once you are comfortable in your peaceful place, invite your Inner Wise Advisor to join you here. Allow an image to form that represents your inner guide. This is a wise and kind figure who

knows you well and wants your greatest good. Let it appear in any way that it shows up—as a woman or man, animal, someone you know, a spiritual figure, a character from a movie or book, or your own Wise Self or Higher Self.

o   Start by asking your Advisor's name. When you are ready, ask any questions you have regarding your purpose; for example, how to serve your purpose in a way that is truly aligned, fulfilling, and impactful. You might ask about any steps you can take toward discovering or serving your purpose. Ask just one question at a time. After asking a question, pause to listen to your Advisor's response. You may hear your Advisor speaking with you or you may experience a felt sense or symbol of their message. Allow the communication to flow in whatever way feels most natural. If you are uncertain about the feedback you receive, feel free to ask more questions to gain clarity. Continue the conversation until you feel you have learned what you can at this time. When the conversation feels complete (for now), thank your Advisor, and if you like, discuss plans to meet again. As you part, your Advisor may have a final gift or message to give you. Allow yourself to receive this. Say goodbye, let your peaceful place fade away, and come back to the present, back to the room where you are seated.

o   Write down anything you learned from this conversation. Imagine what life would be like and how you would feel if you followed the suggestions of your Advisor. Are there any actions you want to take, based on this experience?

Finding and serving our purpose not only brings meaning but also authentic fulfillment. In the next chapter, I will delve deeper into the topic of fulfillment and emotional well-being. I explore how vegan values, along with plant-powered nutrition and healthy lifestyle practices, can contribute to emotional well-being, resilience, and authentic, wholehearted flourishing.

CHAPTER 5

CREATE AUTHENTIC FULFILLMENT

"Becoming fully human is about living a full existence, not one that is continually happy. Being well is not always about feeling good; it also involves continually incorporating more meaning, engagement, and growth in one's life—key themes in humanistic psychology."

—**Scott Barry Kaufman**, in *Transcend: The New Science of Self-Actualization* [1]

"Only those who have learned the power of sincere and selfless contribution experience life's deepest joy: true fulfillment."

—**Tony Robbins**

The desire for happiness drives many of our behaviors. Consider what we buy, the activities we engage in, the relationships we cultivate, and the goals we seek, all in the pursuit of happiness. Yet, defining happiness is not an easy task, nor is achieving it. As individuals, we each have our own take on what constitutes "happiness." Some see happiness as the uplifting emotional state we experience when life is going well, while others equate happiness with a larger sense of overall fulfillment and well-being.

In the field of positive psychology, which studies "what makes life most worth living,"[2] *happiness* is often defined as experiencing a balance of more positive feelings than negative feelings, or by high life satisfaction.[3] Happiness researcher Dr. Sonja Lyubomirsky, author of *The How of Happiness*, describes happiness as "the experience of joy, contentment, or positive well-being, combined with a sense that one's life is good, meaningful, and worthwhile."[4]

However, many researchers argue that "happiness" per se does not fully capture the complexity of human thriving, and that terms such as *well-being* and *fulfillment* may be better descriptors of a life well lived. Martin Seligman, Ph.D., who is often considered "the father of positive psychology," argues that the popular perception of happiness is "inextricably bound up with being in a cheerful mood."[5] He says that this view of happiness "consigns the 50 percent of the world's population who are 'low-positive affectives' to the hell of unhappiness." He goes on to explain, "Even though they lack cheerfulness, this low-mood half may have more engagement and meaning in life than merry people."[6] In other words, many of us may not fit common conceptions of happiness because we are not bubbly, outgoing, or cheerful types. However, we still may experience a sense of meaning and contribution that brings an authentic fulfillment to our lives.

These concerns led Dr. Seligman to shift his focus from his "authentic happiness" theory[7] to studying how we can maximize *emotional well-being* and *flourishing*. He describes emotional well-being as being made up of five core components: *positive emotions* (which include happiness, contentment, and life satisfaction); *engagement* (a sense of being in flow); positive *relationships* (fulfilling connections with others); *meaning* (belonging to and serving something bigger than the self); and *accomplishment* (mastery and achievement). Seligman uses the acronym PERMA to help remember these elements. His research emphasizes that a *combination* of these factors contributes to a life that is fulfilling and flourishing, rather than positive moods alone.[8]

Positive emotions *do* play an important role in our well-being. For example, they appear to open our minds to new experiences, broaden and expand our awareness, lead us to seek and explore, and strengthen our emotional resources.[9] Research shows that experiencing more positive emotions is associated with greater physical and emotional well-being, better relationships, longevity, resilience, and stress reduction.[10]

Positive emotions are naturally reinforcing, and we tend to seek and pursue activities and experiences that heighten them. However, an overfocus on *solely* positive emotions misses the complexity, richness, and fullness of a meaningful, fulfilling (and realistic) human existence. Some discussions on happiness (and how to become happier) overemphasize our own personal agency in creating happiness, while ignoring the impact of societal, cultural, economic, and structural forces that can have a huge impact on how people rate their level of happiness.[11] For example, the Ipsos Global Happiness study of 2019 indicated that, on average, 64 percent of people worldwide reported being "rather happy" or "very happy"; however, this percentage differed greatly from country to country, ranging from 86 percent in Australia and Canada to 34 percent in Argentina.[12]

In addition, researchers have found that experiencing a *variety* of emotions, both positive and negative, is linked to greater overall well-being than experiencing mostly positive emotions. They refer to this range of emotions as *emodiversity* and found that those who reported greater emodiversity experienced less depression and better health. The researchers postulate that perhaps these benefits occur because experiencing a range of different emotions has adaptive value for our survival and thriving. It also may be an indicator of emotional self-awareness and authenticity, both of which have been linked to emotional and physical well-being.[13]

The concept of *eudaimonia*, originally described by Aristotle, embodies a meaningful, purposeful life that is aligned with values and virtues. Aristotle argued that true happiness comes from realizing our potential and contributing to something beyond ourselves. Eudaimonic happiness contrasts with *hedonic* happiness, which focuses primarily on pleasure, enjoyment, and fulfilling desires.[14] Research on what contributes to a fulfilling life is consistent with the concept of eudaimonia. Recent studies found that core contributors to a fulfilling life were being one's true and authentic self, contributing in ways that feel worthwhile and meaningful, and having a positive impact and legacy.[15]

In reality, we need both eudaimonic and hedonic well-being. We need to feel a sense of deeper meaning, and at the same time we need a balance of pleasure and play. A fulfilling life involves a range of emotions, both positive and negative. It includes moments of joy, contentment, and happiness, often fueled by our involvement in activities, relationships, values, and causes that matter to us. It also includes allowing, accepting, and making meaning of our more difficult feelings and experiences. It entails a balance of being and doing. It is an integration of heart, mind, body, and spirit.

As a psychologist who has worked with clients through difficult life experiences and complex emotions, I resonate with this more nuanced understanding of emotional well-being and fulfillment, versus an emphasis on "happiness" as the be-all and end-all. My experience has taught me that we need to experience the full tapestry of our emotions for a full and healthy life. Even the emotions that we label as "negative," like fear, sadness, or anger, serve important adaptive and survival functions, helping us to recognize our needs and to take appropriate action. Many times, we wish to bury or push away negative emotions because we fear becoming overwhelmed by them. However, learning to recognize, acknowledge, and move through our emotions is essential to psychological, physical, and interpersonal wellness. This mindful and self-compassionate acknowledgement of our emotional experience reduces the risk that we will bury our feelings or become "stuck" in a particular emotion. Ultimately, it allows us to engage in life more fully and authentically.

Veganism and fulfillment

This description of an authentic and holistic emotional well-being (which includes a diverse range of emotions) also proved to be highly relevant in understanding the emotional experiences of my vegan research participants. When asked about the ways that veganism contributed to their emotional well-being, the most commonly endorsed responses fit well with positive psychology principles, including alignment with core values, greater meaning and purpose, increased compassion, and meaningful relationships (topics covered in other chapters in this book). In addition, relevant to this chapter's topic, two-thirds of participants reported increased *personal fulfillment* associated with being vegan. Many also described *positive emotions* such as greater peace (70 percent) and happiness (52 percent).

Capturing the full emotional experience of those living a vegan lifestyle can be complex and multifaceted. Vegans may experience a diverse range of emotions, including joy and fulfillment from improving their health, aligning with their values, and contributing to a greater purpose, while at the same time experiencing sadness and anger associated with realizing the detrimental impact of animal agriculture and other exploitative industries. In addition, because veganism is still a minority lifestyle, vegans may experience a lack of understanding from others around them—which, in turn, can impact their emotional state. On top of this, as vegans we are not immune to the "normal" challenges and stressors of everyday life. Thriving emotionally involves appreciating the many positives of vegan living and learning to navigate the complexities, while staying true to one's own values, convictions, and holistic well-being.

As we've noted previously, the decision to be vegan is more than a dietary choice. While food choices are an important aspect of vegan living, choosing to be vegan is also a commitment to deeper values. Whether one chooses veganism for health, ethics, or environmental reasons, it takes dedication to change one's lifestyle and swim against the tide of old habits and societal norms. For many vegans, especially those who sustain the vegan lifestyle over time, veganism becomes a part of their identity that represents their commitment to certain values and ideals. This commitment can contribute to deep and authentic fulfillment for many vegans, as shown in the sampling of survey responses here:

"Veganism is not an elimination diet; it is a lifestyle filled with happiness, peace, and contentment. I love being vegan. I am happy, I am at peace. I live my life to do the most good, while causing the least harm to all living creatures."

"My baseline is now happiness, joy, and contentment. Bad things still happen and affect me, but there is a happiness that underlies everything."

"Sometimes the joy I feel in being vegan makes me want to burst with happiness. [I feel] contentment and peace, knowing that I'm connected to all."

"My confidence level has gone up. I feel more confident in being me."

"My whole life has transformed—truer, freer, and more compassionate. My health has transformed, and I feel like I got my life back."

"I have become more content and accepting of myself. I now like me. I have greater feelings of my own self-worth, significantly better health, and a feeling that I am making a positive difference."

Beyond the personal fulfillment of aligning with vegan values, some survey participants also reported improvement in mental health issues such as anxiety and depression, following their transition to a healthy, whole-food vegan diet, as shown in these responses:

"The most positive changes have been having more mental clarity to be able to do the work to heal and create a life in which I can be more in alignment with who I am meant to be. Emotionally, I have found freedom from mood issues such as anxiety and depression. I feel more clarity with my thinking and connection with my higher power and intuition. I have more compassion for animals and the world, and feel more in alignment with my values and ethics."

"I now have decreased anxiety and depression, increased intuition, purpose, and meaning, and live true to my values. I feel more in tune with who I really am, and much more connected to the energy of the world around me. I am a Reiki practitioner, and my practice has really deepened as I have cleaned up my diet. I also have much more awareness of my emotions and can meditate more deeply."

Societally, the impact of food choices and nutrition on our mental and emotional health is often overlooked. In a culture of fast food, processed food, and heavy reliance on meat and dairy, along with confusing and conflicting information about nutrition, it's easy to feel like we don't have much choice or power in this arena. However, research suggests that nutrient-dense plant foods not only nurture physical health and protect from disease, but also support our emotional thriving. To maximize our fulfillment and emotional well-being, we need to consider the food we put into our bodies. Next, I discuss research on food and emotional health.

Food and Mood

When it comes to improving our *physical health*, there is a vast body of empirical support showing the benefits of a whole-food, vegan diet. As I will discuss in more depth in Chapter Seven, plant-based diets (along with other healthy lifestyle changes) have been shown to prevent and even reverse cardiovascular disease, Type 2 diabetes, autoimmune disease, and some forms of cancer.[16] Plant-exclusive diets are free of cholesterol and low in saturated fat, as well as high in fiber, antioxidants, and micronutrients.

Eating a healthy plant-sourced diet has been shown to reverse mild cognitive decline and reduce the risk of Alzheimer's disease.[17] Plant foods are good not only for our body and vascular system, but also for our brain and nervous system. Given the interconnection between mind and body, it is no surprise that healthy plant nutrition optimizes our emotional well-being.

Benefits of fruits and vegetables

How often have we heard that we should eat our fruits and vegetables? Probably we all have heard this—from our parents, grandparents, and others—yet research suggests that most Americans eat significantly less than the recommended five to nine daily servings.[18] However, if we want to improve our emotional and mental health, it may be a good idea to heed Grandma's advice. Numerous studies[19] have found that people who eat more daily servings of fruits and vegetables report greater emotional well-being and life satisfaction, improved mental health, and decreased emotional distress compared to those who eat lesser amounts.[20] Studies suggest that seven to ten daily servings of fruits and veggies may be optimal.[21]

Fruits and veggies may also support us in going beyond emotional wellness to thriving and flourishing. A study of young adults found that those who consumed more servings of fruits and vegetables scored higher on measures of eudaimonic well-being (defined as a sense of purpose in life), creativity, curiosity, and positive affect, compared to those who ate lesser amounts. The study participants also reported higher levels of these positive emotions on the days they ate more fruits and vegetables compared to the days they had lesser amounts.[22]

Our fruit and vegetable consumption appears to predict our future mood states. A study of young adults found that consuming higher amounts of fruits and vegetables predicted a more positive mood the next day.[23] In addition, a longitudinal study of Australian adults, with assessments taken in 2007, 2009, and 2013, found that increased fruit and veggie intake was predictive of greater happiness, life satisfaction, and well-being at later assessments.[24]

Benefits of a plant-based diet

So, now we know that there are substantial emotional benefits from eating a good daily dose of fruits and veggies. But what do we know about the impact of reducing or eliminating animal products on our mental and emotional well-being?

Many sources on the food–mood connection cite the benefits of the Mediterranean diet.[25] Mediterranean diets, while not exclusively plant-sourced, tend to be high in fruits, vegetables, legumes, nuts, and whole grains, and lower in meat consumption. Several studies have found that a Mediterranean diet pattern is associated with lower risk of depression compared to standard, more omnivorous diets.[26] These studies suggest that the benefits for mental health increase with greater intake of fruit, nuts, and legumes, and with reduced consumption of full-fat dairy, meat, fast food, and fried food.[27]

A cross-sectional study found that vegetarians (who do not eat meat but may consume dairy and eggs) demonstrated lower scores on measures of depression, anxiety, and general emotional distress compared to omnivores.[28] Similarly, another study found that vegans (who ate no animal products) reported lower levels of anxiety and stress than omnivores.[29] A recent Turkish survey of vegetarians, vegans, and omnivores found that participants with a meat-free diet reported lower anxiety and depression, less emotional eating, and less uncontrolled eating compared to omnivores.[30]

Randomized controlled trials (RCTs), in which participants are randomly assigned to a specific treatment condition, are considered the gold standard for research, but these are not easy to implement for many real-life phenomena such as dietary patterns. There have been only a few RCTs looking at vegan diets and mental health, and these studies point to the benefits of plant-based diets. In one study, omnivores who were asked to eliminate meat, poultry, and fish had improved mood scores after two weeks on a vegetarian diet compared to control subjects who continued eating meat.[31] In a research study conducted in a corporate setting, participants who were instructed to eat a vegan diet for health and weight loss not only had improved health measures, but also had decreased depression and anxiety and improved emotional well-being compared to participants in a control group who did not change their diet.[32]

In sum, these studies suggest that eating more plant foods, and decreasing intake of animal foods, can positively impact our mood states and emotional well-being.

What is it about eating plants that helps mental health?

Why does a plant-strong diet help mood? Research suggests that the antioxidants in whole plant foods promote a healthy balance of brain-nourishing neurotransmitters.[33] Antioxidants prevent or slow the damage caused by excessive amounts of free radicals, which are unstable molecules that can contribute to cell damage and disease. Our bodies naturally produce some antioxidants, but the majority comes from the food we eat. The vibrant colors of plant foods reflect their antioxidant content; generally, the brighter or darker in color, the more antioxidants.[34] Plant-based foods, seasonings, and beverages, including fruits, berries, vegetables, herbs, spices, and tea, are much richer in antioxidants than animal-based foods.[35]

Antioxidant-rich plant foods have been shown to decrease inflammation, which appears to have a beneficial impact on brain functioning and mood. Inflammation is not always bad; in the short run, inflammation helps our bodies respond to and heal from injuries or illness. However, *chronic* inflammation, often caused or exacerbated by lifestyle factors such as diet, stress, and sedentary behavior, is associated with physical health problems, including heart disease, diabetes, and autoimmune disease,[36] as well as depression.[37] In contrast to the anti-inflammatory effects of plant foods, animal products (i.e., meat, eggs, and dairy) are associated with higher levels of inflammatory compounds,[38] which may negatively impact mental and emotional states.[39]

Dietary fiber, which is found only in plants, not animal foods, is also associated with improved mood and decreased depression.[40] Fiber is the roughage from plants, which helps our digestion and fosters healthy gut bacteria. Researchers are increasingly recognizing the importance of a healthy gut for good mental health. Somewhat surprisingly, the gut provides the vast majority (95 percent) of our body's mood-supporting serotonin.[41] A recent meta-analysis found that with each five gram *increase* in total dietary fiber intake, there was a corresponding five percent *decrease* in risk of depression.[42] This is particularly important given that most Americans consume less than half of the fiber than recommended by the USDA.[43] Simply by increasing our intake of high-fiber foods, we can improve our emotional well-being.

Overall, these studies show that eating a plant-rich diet and reducing or eliminating meat, dairy, and highly processed foods decreases inflammation and may improve mental health. These studies highlight the importance of *quality* nutrition for optimizing brain functioning and emotional well-being; for example, including a variety of colorful fruits and veggies, legumes, nuts, and whole grains. Fiber and antioxidants from plants play a crucial role in our emotional well-being, and, importantly, this appears to occur primarily through whole foods, *not* supplements.[44]

What about those headlines claiming that vegans are depressed?

In recent years, some headlines in popular media have claimed that meatless diets are associated with greater depression and/or anxiety.[45] In trying to make sense of these media headlines, which appear to contradict the extensive research showing benefits of plant-powered diets, I spent a considerable amount of time reading the articles and checking out the studies they referenced. Many media articles focused on summaries of recently published studies, and often did not address nuances, mixed results, or problems with the studies. And some claims were based largely on anecdotal reports.[46]

Some of these headlines were sparked by the conclusions of a research review and meta-analysis on the relationship between meat eating and mental health, conducted by psychology researchers from the University of Southern Indiana.[47] A meta-analysis is a statistical process for examining the data from several studies on a topic and identifying trends and common findings. Meta-analysis can be one of the most robust empirical approaches to research in that it draws on numerous studies on a particular issue. It is not a foolproof type of research, however, and its validity can be eroded by weaknesses in the studies cited and how these studies were selected and interpreted.

Based on their meta-analyses, the researchers concluded that across the studies they examined, the "prevalence or risk of depression and/or anxiety were significantly greater in participants who avoided meat consumption."[48] The authors acknowledged that some studies showed the reverse (greater depression and anxiety in meat-eaters), and some studies had mixed or non-significant findings. They also noted that the cited studies were correlational and therefore did not prove causation. (The only randomized controlled trial showed that participants eating a meat-free diet had more positive mood scores than those consuming meat).[49] This lack of causal relationship was emphasized by one of the initial study's authors, Edward Archer. In a conversation with *Business Insider*, he clarified that the meta-analysis results do not show that meat consumption improves mental health, nor that not consuming meat worsens it.[50]

Closer examination of the meta-analysis highlights several concerns.[51] First, a relatively small number of available studies were ultimately included in the analyses, and most were reported to show some risk of bias. In some studies, semi-vegetarians, vegetarians, and/or vegans were lumped together. There were very few vegans in most studies, which brings into question how representative the findings were for vegans. Most studies did not look at the nutritional quality of the diet, so it's unknown if this would make a difference in outcomes.

In addition, nuances of study results were often overlooked or minimized in the authors' conclusions. For example, one study cited as supporting the benefits of meat-eating found that vegetarian and pescatarian diets were associated with greater depression, but only for those with *low legume* consumption, not those with higher legume intake. This same study found that *low vegetable* consumption was also associated with increased depression in all dietary groups. In addition, after controlling for possible confounding variables, vegan diets were *not* associated with greater depression.[52] Another study referenced in the meta-analysis as supporting omnivorous diets instead highlighted the important role of culture in the relationship between diet and mental health. This study found that vegetarianism was *not* associated with mental health status for US, Russian, or German residents; however, it was associated with slight increases in anxiety and depression in Chinese participants.[53]

Last, but not least, the greatest concern about this study's claims: *The meta-analysis research was funded by the Beef Industry.* At the bottom of the publication, it states, "This study was funded in part via an unrestricted research grant from the Beef Checkoff, through the National Cattlemen's Beef Association. The sponsor of the study had no role in the study design, data collection, data analysis, data interpretation, or writing of the report."[54] As further explained by *Business Insider*, the lead researcher of these papers received a $10,555 grant from the National Cattlemen's Beef Association "to conduct a systematic review on 'Beef for a Happier and Healthier life.'"[55] One must wonder how the researchers' orientation toward this research, and possible bias and/or conflicts of interest associated with the funding source, impacted the meta-analysis study selection, interpretation, and conclusions.[56]

It is important to add that a recent research review by other investigators came to different conclusions. A meta-analysis of 13 studies published in 2022 by Askari et al. found no significant relationship between vegetarianism and depression and anxiety.[57]

One takeaway from my review of the research on diet and mental health is that it is often difficult for research studies to capture the complexity of real life. Cross-sectional studies comparing the mental health of vegetarians, vegans, and omnivores rarely address the complex interplay of diet, nutrition, lifestyle, values, culture, and social context, and how these connect to emotional well-being. And oftentimes, I found that the authors' orientation seemed to reflect the worldview of the status quo (i.e., that meat eating is "natural, normal, and necessary" and that those who do not eat meat must therefore be abnormal or unhealthy). Often, their discussion and framework showed little understanding of the varied reasons people choose a plant-based (meat-free) lifestyle—for personal health, emotional fulfillment, ethics, values alignment, and/or caring for animals and the environment.[58]

Most of these studies do not acknowledge the diverse experiences and motivations of vegans and vegetarians, who choose a meat-free lifestyle for a variety of reasons. For many, veganism goes far beyond being a "diet" to being a lifestyle and an ethical commitment. This commitment to a larger cause, and the increased attunement to cruelty and injustice, an attunement not yet shared by most of society, can bring complex and multifaceted emotions that are not easily assessed or understood in large-scale, cross-sectional studies.

Further, vegans live in diverse cultures and social circumstances, some of which provide support for a plant-based lifestyle, and some of which are relatively unsupportive. Consider the United States, for example, where we are inundated with food advertising, media messages, and social gatherings that emphasize meat and other animal products, with little acknowledgement of the benefits of a plant-based lifestyle. The level of support that we have for our diet and lifestyle (or lack thereof) plays a significant role in our sense of well-being.

To sum this up, many vegans find deep and authentic fulfillment from their vegan lifestyle. It appears that eating nutritious *whole* plant foods (and fewer highly processed foods) provides added benefits of improved brain health and greater emotional well-being. In addition, vegans often describe feeling lighter and more peaceful as they eat life-giving plant foods, and no longer consume the suffering and death inherent in animal foods.

True fulfillment is found when we align in mind, body, and spirit; when we honor our values, nourish our whole self, and engage in what most matters to us. This is the kind of fulfillment that comes with listening to our heart, being receptive to change and growth, and embracing both the gifts and challenges of life. Next I share the stories of two research interviewees whose lives exemplify this type of authentic fulfillment.

Abbie and Lee Nelson are a vegan couple with two young children whom they are raising vegan. They each describe emotional fulfillment and growth during their vegan journeys, even as they deal with the stressors and challenges of being new parents, working, and attending graduate school.

Abbie's story

Abbie was a social work doctoral student at the time of her interview. She indicated that when she was younger, she struggled with mental health issues and an eating disorder. She was an excellent student and athlete, but internally struggled with anxiety and depression. After high school, she sought an undergraduate degree and then a master's degree in social work. She explains that she always had a passion for social justice issues, and over time she gained greater awareness around animal justice issues.

> What finally opened my eyes was my first marriage; I was in a domestic violence relationship. Everything went downhill, along with my mental health and my physical health, and at the same time, I was also getting my clinical licensure and working as a counselor. My life was super stressful, personally and professionally. My body was shot. I had adrenal fatigue; my hormones were screwed up. I was trying to figure out what to do to heal, and of course, the medical model wanted to put me on more meds. So, I went on my own spiritual and emotional journey. I was trying to research what my other options are. Then I came across this tiny little book about a lady who had used a raw vegan diet to help balance and manage emotional symptoms. I felt like, "this is my path!"

Abbie started on a raw vegan diet but didn't have support to transition successfully. She states, "I was really isolated. I didn't know anyone who was vegan. I tried to go from eating lots of meat and cheese to a fully raw vegan diet." After a couple of months, she was not feeling well physically, so she returned to her former way of eating. However, she noted, "My eyes had been opened to realize that this is about more than just health. I now saw the connection to animals."

Abbie continued to learn more about veganism. "I believed in the potential of a vegan diet, but I didn't know how to do it. And I was so stressed out in my life that I thought, 'I can't have one more thing to throw me over the edge.' I just wasn't at a time in my life, honestly, where I had enough emotional energy to make the transition." She enjoyed listening to vegan podcasts, and gradually realized, "This totally aligns with social work. This can help poverty. This can help environmental justice. I started understanding these connections."

Abbie continued taking steps toward a more plant-based lifestyle over the next couple of years. Then in 2017, she divorced her abusive partner, became vegan, and trained for a half-Ironman. She acknowledged that the changes were not easy. But her growing understanding of the larger impacts of a vegan lifestyle helped her to work through the challenges of her transition. She stated, "In the beginning, my decision to go vegan was for me, for my health. When I understood it was also about the world, my clients, and the universe, that's when I could no longer go back."

Abbie made vegan friends, joined vegan groups, and met Lee, who was already vegan. This support helped immensely in adjusting to her new lifestyle. As she became aware of the connection between poor mental health and diet, she sought training as a Vegan Lifestyle Coach and Educator through Main Street Vegan Academy so that she could integrate this knowledge into her work with clients. She was also trained in psychotherapeutic yoga, to bring holistic healing practices to her clients.

In about 2018, after undergoing an extended water fast with her husband, they both shifted to a raw vegan diet. She indicated that subsequently, she noticed less inflammation, reduced "puffiness," and clearer skin. She also reported sleeping better and feeling stronger physically and mentally. She explained:

> It took me a while to get to the place I am now, mentally and spiritually. Initially, when I went vegan, I was detoxing from my old diet and I had brain fog at first. But I was committed and stuck through it. Some time after shifting to a raw vegan diet, my brain fog cleared up. And I could feel, spiritually, that I was more sensitive to my clients. In one way, life became a bit harder for me, because I was so open and clear, all my senses heightened. Sometimes that can be very intense.
>
> I'm able to connect with my higher self in a stronger way. I feel this connection to the world, and sometimes it becomes overwhelming. For example, when we were in quarantine for COVID, it was so overwhelming for me. When I would go into meditation, I could literally feel this global pain. And I feel that sometimes with the animals. I'll see a transport truck that carries the animals and literally have a hard time breathing. I can feel the oppression.
>
> I'm an empath, and I always had this capacity. But back when I was addicted to food, and food was a drug to me, it kind of numbed

these things. I'm a therapist myself, but I've still had to seek help on how to manage my energy and manage this openness that I now have. I can't go around all day feeling that intensity—I have to be able to contain it. But I do think my ability to connect with humanity and all life is a gift. I can touch a tree and feel it pulsing with me. I think we all have this ability, but our life is so rushed. You know, we're covered up with chemicals. It's a gift that being a raw vegan can bring.

I'm more aligned with who I'm meant to be in this world. And that doesn't always equate with happiness. I'm focused on, "How do I live the most meaningful life?" To me, that's having the rainbow of emotions. There have been times in my life where I didn't have enough emotional resilience to allow myself to be able to feel these feelings. But I did a lot of inner work. I don't think that it's just the food alone that contributes to well-being. While I was changing my diet, I was also doing therapy, meditation, and yoga to prepare myself to live this lifestyle. It's not just a diet, it's definitely a lifestyle. I want to be a part of shifting humanity toward healing and hope. I feel that this is a big part of doing that, living this lifestyle, and sharing this with other people. There's so much we need to be doing. But this is one way toward creating positive change. Even on days when there is so much going on that all I can do is make it through the day, it's grounding to know that this lifestyle I'm choosing is helping the world today.

Abbie stated that, through her vegan journey, she found empowerment in her emotional and mental health. Her experience has led her to explore the benefits of a plant-based diet for survivors of domestic violence as part of her doctoral research. She said, "My ultimate goal is to develop a plant-based protocol along with psychotherapy. I recognize the need to support survivors in a holistic way. Most treatment approaches don't include the diet at all. We cannot deny that what our clients are putting in their body is affecting how they're showing up in this world. When you're eating meat, you're eating dead beings. You're literally putting pain, violence, and oppression in your body. Choosing to eat plants brings life and healing."

Lee's story

Abbie's husband, Lee, works as a health coach and for an environmental advocacy group. For him, a vegan lifestyle has been an integral part of his journey to greater emotional and spiritual fulfillment.

Lee grew up on a dairy farm. He noted, "I had no examples in my life of vegetarians or vegans. The way that I grew up, I learned that you had to eat meat and dairy products in order to survive. Now looking back from the standpoint of a vegan, I realize that I was so disconnected. I had such a great love for the animals, and then I would go home and eat them."

He indicated that he became interested in health and fitness after working with a chiropractor who recommended stretching exercises. Lee started playing softball, soccer, and working out. He was told by fellow athletes that if he wanted to bulk up, he needed to eat more protein; specifically, more meat. He started eating more meat, but "it didn't work. I didn't get big; I didn't gain a lot of muscle. And I started feeling crappy. I wondered, 'What is going on?'"

I had a breaking point one evening when I was cooking ground beef on the stove. The aroma of it, the smell, overwhelmed me. And I started having this emotional response, feeling the emotions of the cows. I think part of it was because of my connection with cows when growing up on a dairy farm. I realized I don't want to eat this. Pretty soon after that, I became pescatarian. I ate fish and some dairy products. I still didn't have anyone around me who was vegetarian or vegan. I just knew that eating all that meat wasn't working. Not too long after that, I started dating a girl who was vegetarian. I also started getting into vinyasa yoga and did yoga teacher training to become a teacher myself. I later did Reiki training, and it was during that training when I transitioned to vegan. I didn't know what I was doing. I just wanted to eat super clean. I thought I would just do it for three months during the training, and then I would go back, because my whole life I drank huge amounts of milk each day. But after a couple weeks, I thought, "I don't want it anymore. I have no desire to go back."

I started doing some research. I wondered how to do this in the healthiest way possible. I came across Dr. Doug Graham, a raw vegan, who wrote the book *The 80/10/10 Diet*, and went to one of his retreats. At this retreat, there were a couple of other older guys, who were in their late sixties. And they're running around like teenagers. And then there were these young girls in their twenties. They had perfect skin, and they're doing these ultra marathons—crazy, amazing things. I thought, "This is what I want right here." It took me a couple years to transition from eating cooked vegan foods to being mostly raw. There was a transition period, and a detox initially. It's been over eight years now that I've been vegan. And I have gone back and forth between being fully raw and sometimes incorporating some cooked foods, like potatoes. I will never compromise on being vegan, but to eat some cooked (vegan) food is not a big issue for me. Being fully raw can be intense from an emotional and spiritual sense.

In the past, I had a lot of issues with feeling emotions in general. I had a tendency to not feel, and so for me, it's been an interesting growth experience to feel emotions more deeply. I think it's helped me to connect with myself, to know myself better. Yoga training and meditation helped me to get to know my mind. Through my training, I learned that raw fruits have the highest energetic vibration. That really aligned for me.

One of the biggest reasons I continue this diet and lifestyle is because I'm honoring my higher self, and my morals and values. It's being in alignment with my environment, with the earth, and with the animals. I've had more spiritual experiences in nature with animals now after becoming vegan. I experience nature in a completely different way. It's a much deeper experience. When I go into nature, I'm aware that nature is responding to me. It's almost like I had blinders on before and now they're off. I just go for a walk, and I feel the experience of the plants around me and of the air and the energy that I'm in. It's beautiful and magical.

There is a big sadness, when I look back into my past, because I did have connections with the cows on our dairy farm and I can see times when I wasn't very nice to them. I can see how eating meat would trigger certain things in me, and I would be angry or lash out or be mean to animals. Even though that wasn't my true self, and I can see that now. I try to have grace for myself and forgive myself and do what I can to promote compassion now.

As far as emotional and spiritual, I believe that a vegan diet and lifestyle can be a great support, but we still have to do the work, whether that's to get therapy, meditate, do breathing exercises, anything to increase self-awareness. The diet alone won't heal or fix everything. I believe this lifestyle is a great support because when I am in alignment with my true self, making decisions that support life, I have more confidence in myself and how I show up in the world, and I can work with more grace through the healing and becoming journey.

The stories of Abbie and Lee, and many other vegans whom I interviewed, demonstrate how a vegan lifestyle can pave the way to personal fulfillment that is centered on authenticity, wholeness, holistic well-being, and a greater appreciation for the natural world. Their stories also highlight how we can enjoy the full spectrum of our emotional experience when we no longer eat foods that deaden our senses and our compassion.

Action Steps

Becoming authentically fulfilled is about whole-life healing and well-being. It encompasses your heart, mind, body, and spirit. The following are action steps to deepen your well-being and fulfillment on your plant-powered journey. Select the actions that most resonate with you.

- **Start by clarifying what *fulfillment* means to you.** Consider these reflection questions to help you explore this. Write your responses in your journal.
    o   What type of person do you most want to be?
    o   What qualities would you exhibit in your most fulfilled life?
    o   What activities, relationships, and values mean the most to you?
    o   When do you currently feel most fulfilled? How can you strengthen these activities, qualities, and experiences in your life?
    o   What is missing or neglected that you want to build or strengthen?
    o   What is one action you can take toward greater fulfillment?
- **Enjoy nourishing plant-sourced meals.** Increase your emotional well-being through healthy, wholesome foods. Focus on both nutritional quality AND enjoyment. Include these mood-boosting foods and nutrients (based on the recommendations of Dr. Neal Barnard and registered dietician Ginny Messina).[59] *Track your mood, coping, and mental focus, and notice how you respond to different foods.*

- Legumes, including beans, chickpeas, lentils, tofu, tempeh, and/or hummus. Protein-rich legumes are high in tryptophan, which is a precursor for serotonin, a neurotransmitter that helps boost mood.
- Plenty of fruits and vegetables, aiming for as much variety as possible. Strive for seven to ten servings per day.
- High-fiber foods. This includes most plant foods: beans, fruits, veggies, nuts and seeds, and whole grains (e.g., oatmeal, brown rice, quinoa, farro).
- Vitamin B-12, which is essential for a healthy brain and nervous system. Some foods are fortified with it, but most physicians recommend B-12 supplementation to ensure adequate intake—about 2.4 mcg per day.[60]
- If you live in a location where you don't get much sunshine, many physicians recommend Vitamin D supplementation.
- Get your essential Omega-3s through flax seeds, chia seeds, hemp seeds, walnuts, and/or plant- or algae-based supplements. Avoid the saturated fat, mercury, and toxins often found in fish or fish oil, and go straight to the original plant sources.

- **What lifestyle practices support your emotional well-being?** What do you currently do to nurture yourself? What new practices might be helpful for greater life balance and well-being? Consider the following:
  - Meditation, mindfulness practices, or yoga
  - Exercise and fun activities that get you moving
  - Adequate rest and sleep
  - Enjoyable interests and hobbies
  - Time with loved ones
  - Spiritual practices
  - Journaling and self-reflection
  - Experiences that bring joy, play, and laughter

- **Cultivate gratitude and awe.** What we focus on has a big impact on our level of fulfillment. Consider the following suggestions for deepening your awareness of the gifts, blessings, beauty, and wonder around you:

o   Spend regular time in nature, and mindfully notice your surroundings, using all your senses. Whether visiting a park, hiking in a forest, walking in your neighborhood, or traveling to a beautiful destination, time in nature is healing for us emotionally.[61] It helps us get out of our heads and reconnect with what is important, experiencing the beauty, majesty, and awesomeness of the planet upon which we live, and the mystery of the galaxies beyond. It also reminds us of the importance of caring for our planet and its inhabitants, and the consequences when we do not.

o   Spend time with animals, whether your own companion animals, or visiting shelters or sanctuaries. Time with non-human animals is healing and nurtures our emotional well-being.

o   If you are vegan, take time each day to notice the blessings of your vegan lifestyle. How has it positively impacted you emotionally, physically, and/or spiritually? How does your vegan lifestyle positively affect others around you? How does it influence your relationship with animals and with nature? Even though there is still much suffering around us, how does being vegan make a positive difference?

- **Create your Authentic Fulfillment action plan.** Review your journal responses and the preceding suggestions. Choose a few actions or lifestyle practices that you want to implement. Create a plan, setting times in your calendar to remind you to follow through.

As you explore what brings greater fulfillment to your own life, one important ingredient that can't be overlooked is the quality of your relationships. Building meaningful, nurturing, and supportive relationships is integral to a healthy and fulfilling life, and to a thriving vegan lifestyle. The next chapter dives into this important topic.

CHAPTER 6

THE POWER OF TRUE CONNECTION

"The desire for love and intimacy is a basic human need, as fundamental as eating, breathing, or sleeping—and the consequences of ignoring that need are just as dire."
—**Dean Ornish**, M.D., in *Love & Survival* [1]

"The greatness of a community is most accurately measured by the compassionate actions of its members."
—**Coretta Scott King**

It was 2007, early on my veg journey. I had just stayed up much of the night reading *The Food Revolution* by John Robbins.[2] I was haunted by the stories and statistics—about immense animal suffering, human health crises, and environmental destruction caused by our food choices. I was learning about factory farming—the overcrowding of animals, the horrific conditions in which they live, and the industrialized slaughter process that treats sentient beings like products in a disassembly line.

There was no one in my immediate social circle whom I could talk to about what I was learning (except for my significant other, who, thankfully, listened to my impassioned rants with the patience of Job). No one else understood the gravity of the situation or seemed willing to talk about any of this. Everyone around me was doing what I used to do—mindlessly eating the Standard American Diet, heavy in meat, dairy, eggs, sweets, and processed foods. It felt like no one wanted to hear anything that might disrupt their customary eating patterns.

I was at Starbucks with a friend from my church, a devoted vegan. We sat down with our beverages, my friend requesting plant-based milk rather than cow's milk. I expressed my distress in realizing the billions of animals slaughtered each year, and the unspeakable suffering in how they are raised and ultimately killed. I was also grappling with learning about the environmental impact—deforestation, the depletion of land and water, pollution, carbon emissions, and the destruction of ecosystems. I wondered how I hadn't seen this or known this before. All this new awareness seemed heavier because I had to carry it largely alone.

As I poured out my feelings, my friend's presence and understanding were very reassuring. I don't remember much of what we said, just that our time together was a comforting balm amid my disillusionment and distress. She had experienced similar emotions when she made these discoveries and came to the same realizations years ago. She understood what I was feeling.

After that supportive visit with my vegan friend, I continued to read and learn about the impacts of my food choices. What I learned strengthened my commitment, and I moved from daily meat eater to mostly vegetarian, to fully vegetarian, and, in time, to vegan. At every stage of my journey, finding support from others who were undergoing the same journey was key to not only sustaining my lifestyle, but also being a fulfilled and thriving vegan.

I met other vegans through a local veg group, which offered educational meetings, social gatherings, and restaurant outings. There was something very special about sharing a plant-based meal and conversation with others who were committed to similar values. I was also amazed by the virtual connections I formed with vegans across the globe, all sharing my passion for creating a kinder, healthier, and more sustainable world. These conversations and communities were like a warm embrace, inspiring and uplifting me, and engaging me in a global movement of compassion and justice for all beings.

These vegan supports helped me gain confidence to speak up in situations where I was the only vegan. When I first became vegan, I was unsure how to navigate typical social gatherings with my non-vegan family and friends. Even though I was strongly committed to my new lifestyle, I found it difficult to explain the changes in my diet or to even utter the "V" word. I was still processing all that I was learning, and not yet ready for possible judgment, questioning, or confrontation. I was caught up in an inner conflict between "not rocking the boat," and honoring my truth. Gradually, through talking to vegan friends and reading books by vegan authors, I learned to be proactive and prepared for handling social situations. Also, rather than viewing my new dietary requirements as an inconvenience to myself or others, I realized that my needs and values were worthy of being expressed and honored.

I found the courage to begin speaking up, asking for what I needed, explaining what veganism is, and why I am vegan. I became better at sharing this in ways that elicited curiosity and conversation rather than contention. To my surprise, I found that most people were incredibly supportive, especially when I expressed myself in a heartfelt way. I also learned that it is not a bad thing for disagreement or differing views to arise; I discovered that working through them often contributes to lively conversations and a more robust mutual understanding and connection. And sometimes, it even leads to transformation—in me, in the other person, and in our relationship.[3]

Connecting through vegan values

There is something incredibly meaningful about connecting with like-minded (and like-hearted) others who have common values, concerns, and passions. Similar to what I experienced with my vegan friend at the coffee shop, sharing our feelings and concerns with people who understand where we are coming from provides affirmation and sustenance. We feel connected and less alone. Our shared experiences and convictions reinforce that connection. Finding a caring and like-minded community brings nourishment and inspiration.

These kinds of supportive relationships were highlighted again and again by the participants in my research. "Connecting with others who share my values" was reported by my survey respondents to be one of the most emotionally fulfilling aspects of being vegan. Many respondents were involved in vegan groups or organizations, and some were even founders or leaders of these organizations. Through the shared passion of veganism, they found authentic personal connections that made them feel understood and supported. This support and understanding provided a foundation for collaboration and contribution to a common cause. The survey responses that follow illustrate these meaningful connections:

"I have connected with other like-minded people and have more meaningful relationships than ever before."

"I created a virtual world of like-minded individuals I can start to call friends. I found a Tribe and it feels great."

"I've met so many wonderful, compassionate people since becoming vegan. It has helped me focus where I volunteer my time (e.g., animal sanctuaries), where I donate, and helps me live a life of purpose."

"I feel a sense of freedom in living in sync with my values. This has led me to pursue a different career path and build community with like-minded people . . . I have described going vegan as feeling like I came home."

"I met an amazing set of beautiful souls who have the same purpose in life. I have been blessed to be associated with an organization that resonates with my values and catalyzes my connection in this serene space. The fact that there are authentic, credible, and inspirational people who are so much into this that their entire life and work revolves around this is very reassuring."

"My activism often pushes me out of my comfort zone and leads me to interact with other people more. My social skills have gotten better as a result, and I'm much more able to push through whatever anxiety I'm feeling, knowing that this is so much more important."

Our need for community

Healthy and supportive relationships are paramount to our emotional and physical well-being. As noted in the opening quote by Dean Ornish, our need for connection and intimacy is as basic as our physiological needs for air, water, and food. Most of us intuitively know this, and science has backed up how important it is for us to have a sense of connection, belonging, and intimacy with others.[4] The longest scientific study on happiness, the Harvard Study of Adult Development, has followed the same individuals and their families since 1938 to investigate what contributes to a happy and healthy life, drawing on in-depth interviews, medical evaluations, brain scans, and blood work.[5] In his 2015 TEDx talk, Dr. Robert Waldinger, the study's current lead investigator, summarizes the findings: "Well, the lessons aren't about wealth or fame or working harder and harder. The clearest message we get from this 75-year study is this: Good relationships keep us happier and healthier. Period."[6]

According to Waldinger, the results show that healthy relationships are associated with better happiness, physical health, and longevity, while isolation and loneliness negatively impact physical and emotional health. He explains that it is not so much the *number* of connections that matters; rather, the *quality* of relationships and one's satisfaction with their relationships are key in predicting future health and longevity. Conversely, toxic relationships have a detrimental effect on health.[7]

It seems that everywhere you look, there is more research supporting the vital importance of quality relationships for our physical and emotional well-being. I was surprised to learn that loneliness and lack of social support are as detrimental to our health and longevity as smoking, obesity, high blood pressure, and physical inactivity.[8] Loneliness and isolation increase the risk of premature death and are associated with higher risk of heart disease, stroke, and dementia. In addition, those with greater loneliness are more likely to experience anxiety, depression, and/or suicidal ideation.[9] The importance of quality relationships to our overall well-being makes sense intuitively, and it is enlightening to learn from empirical studies just how essential they are.

Dr. Dean Ornish, who is perhaps best known for his revolutionary research on preventing and reversing heart disease, emphasizes the importance of healthy relationships for protecting our health. His Lifestyle Medicine program, which incorporates plant-based nutrition, physical exercise, smoking cessation, relaxation skills, and group support, has been scientifically shown to reverse cardiovascular disease. Vascular imaging studies showed visible improvements in patients' previously blocked arteries after following his protocol.[10] Notwithstanding the crucial role of diet and nutrition in healing chronic disease, Dr. Ornish states that the importance of relationships is often overlooked. In his book *Love & Survival*, he argued that "love and intimacy are among the most powerful factors in health and illness, even though these ideas are largely ignored by the medical profession."[11]

Researchers argue that from an evolutionary standpoint, forming strong social bonds has helped humanity to survive and thrive through millennia. Social support and acceptance are so central to our well-being that when we feel excluded or rejected, we experience similar distress to that caused by bodily pain. In fact, research by social psychologist Dr. Naomi Eisenberger has shown that the experience of social loss and rejection lights up the same brain regions as physical pain. She explains that this connection between social and physical pain might play a protective role; when we feel the threat of social loss, the associated distress motivates us to heal or guard our social connections.[12] We appear to be equipped with a highly sensitive social protection system that guides us to detect and respond to any threats to our social belonging.[13]

As noted earlier, the *quality* of our connections is integral to our emotional and physical well-being. Relationship researchers distinguish between low-quality and high-quality connections. To get a sense of how this works in real life, take a moment to reflect on different relational experiences you have had. First, think about experiences when you didn't feel connected with the other person. Maybe they weren't emotionally present, or there was lingering unresolved conflict or hostility, or indifference, or a lack of common ground. Whatever the cause, you may have found yourself feeling depleted, drained, and/or more isolated after this encounter. Contrast this with high-quality relational experiences, in which you felt deeply engaged, energized, nourished, and supported. These kinds of high-quality connections are typically grounded in a sense of safety and security, feeling that the other person has our back, along with being connected, understood, and valued.[14] Engagement in high-quality connections fosters positive shared experiences, energy and vitality, mutual give-and-take, and a sense of unconditional positive regard.[15]

We feel a special sense of well-being when we are in community with others who share our concerns and values. These common bonds provide the foundation for meaningful connection. When we bond around a shared passion, commitment, concern, or cause, it provides numerous benefits. For one, we no longer feel alone. There is great relief and comfort in connecting with others who share our views, challenges, and joys. In addition, these kindred supports cheer us on and give us encouragement. They can be a source of assistance and guidance when we have difficulties, and they provide camaraderie, collaboration, inspiration, and synergy. As noted earlier, this type of energizing connection among fellow vegans was described by my vegan participants as one of the aspects of veganism that they found most fulfilling.

Finding a like-minded community may be especially important when we are dealing with anything that makes us different than most people around us. The Blue Zones, geographic locations where people live the longest and healthiest lives (referenced previously in Chapter Four), highlight that fellowship with people who share our values and lifestyle is crucial. Having an aligned community, what Blue Zones researcher Dan Buettner calls "Right Tribe," reinforces and supports the types of behaviors we want to maintain.[16]

The normative behaviors in our social networks tend to be contagious (for better or for worse). Research finds that people are likely to follow the common trends and habits of their social network. Our social groups can have a major influence on whether we eat a healthy diet, exercise, and/or use unhealthy substances. Therefore, if we want to live a lifestyle that defies the status quo, we greatly benefit from the support of others who are on the same path.[17]

Social support for your vegan journey

Given the importance of healthy connections who support and encourage us on our vegan path, we need to be mindful of our social resources. Since veganism is currently a minority lifestyle, the need for aligned support is essential. In fact, research suggests that social barriers are primary triggers for lapsing from veganism. For example, the desire to fit in socially and not inconvenience others was cited as a reason that some stray from their plant-based lifestyle.[18] Having a strong social network with other vegans appears to strengthen commitment and adherence to a vegan lifestyle.[19]

To experience the mind-body-spirit transformation that is possible with a vegan lifestyle, we can't do it alone. We need others we can talk to, to share our travails, hopes and dreams, challenges, and daily experiences. We need others to walk the journey with us. Others who understand what we feel and encourage us when we are down. Others who will collaborate with us toward a shared vision, whether to be more fit and healthy, awaken spiritually, advocate for animals, fight for social justice, or work toward environmental and climate healing. These collaborative and supportive relationships inspire, uplift, and nurture us. They give us hope and strengthen our commitment during challenging times.

Here lies one of the paradoxes of the vegan experience. On one hand, as vegans we have discovered truths that deeply impact everything we care about—and this often leads to meaningful connections with others who share the same concerns and vision. This shared commitment fosters high-quality connections that may be beyond what we have ever experienced before. But on the other hand, we may feel disconnected or isolated when family and friends are not interested in learning about a vegan or plant-based lifestyle or understanding why it matters to us.

Participants in my survey research acknowledged that social challenges were common. About two-thirds reported that they've experienced a lack of support or understanding from others in their life who are not vegan. Nearly half indicated that they had at some point been ridiculed for being vegan, and around 40 percent reported that at times they felt left out or excluded in social situations.

Learning to strengthen supportive connections with other vegans as well as with non-vegan friends and family is a core skill displayed by fulfilled and thriving vegans. This skill is learnable, and it is transformative. Many of my survey respondents noted that, although they experienced social difficulties early in their vegan journey, they learned how to cope with and/or overcome many of these challenges over time. As expressed by one survey respondent, "I have become more independent in my thinking, less likely to succumb to fearing the opinions of others, less affected by trying to fit in, less likely to worry about being judged by prevailing social attitudes."

The following are five common factors that my vegan participants found helpful for building greater social fulfillment and connection:

1. **Seeking support from other vegans**. The most fulfilled vegans were actively involved in vegan groups or networks, whether participating in online meetings or classes, going to local meetups,

running a vegan business, or volunteering for a vegan or animal rights organization. They sought out and cultivated like-minded vegan friendships in which they felt supported, nurtured, inspired, and connected. They had safe spaces with other vegans where they could share feelings and concerns, ask for help and guidance to deal with challenges, and work toward a shared vision. It wasn't the size of the network that was most important; having even a few vegan friends often made a huge difference in feeling supported and connected.

2. **Being okay with being different**. This is a big one—because for many people, it isn't easy to go against the status quo. As noted earlier in the chapter, we are biologically wired to need social connections and to want to avoid social exclusion or rejection. Some people are more naturally rebellious and may not find this as difficult, but for many, it can be a major struggle. Thriving vegans discover how to shift their mindset around the idea of being "different." They remember their reasons for choosing a vegan lifestyle so that they can hold their beliefs in the face of social pressures. They learn how to speak up and honor their values in ways that also nurture close connections with others. And at the same time, they realize that not everyone is in the same place on the journey. They come to see that they are early adopters of a movement for health, compassion, and planetary healing, and that being an early adopter and daring to make choices outside the status quo takes courage and integrity.

3. **Learning to speak up assertively and effectively**. Thriving vegans develop the ability to express their feelings, needs, and perspectives in ways that create heartfelt dialogue. Unfortunately, many people lack the ability to skillfully navigate differences, and this leads to unresolved conflicts and emotional cut-offs. Those who thrive as vegans work to develop healthy communication skills so that they can effectively explain veganism to others, patiently respond to repeated questions, and express their feelings and needs. They set boundaries around which situations they are willing (or not willing) to be part of and discover new ways to connect with those they love, including altering or replacing old traditions that center around animal foods.

4. **Creating vegan allies**. To thrive as a vegan, it is very helpful when those closest to us (partners, immediate family) are on board with our lifestyle. However, even when loved ones are not ready or willing to be plant-based themselves, thriving vegans learn to create an environment that supports their lifestyle. They specifically request what they need from their loved ones and clarify what is helpful and what is not. In her book *Beyond Beliefs*, Dr. Melanie Joy emphasizes the value of cultivating vegan "allies" who understand and support our vegan choice. These are people who, although not necessarily vegan themselves, do not undermine our choice to be vegan and advocate for us when we need support.[20]

5. **Planting seeds for positive change**. Thriving vegans focus on being positive role models who embody the compassion, ethics, and well-being they wish to inspire in others. Rather than staying stuck in frustration when others are not willing to change, they realize that everyone has their own journey, and that pressuring or judging others rarely works to create personal or social transformation. At the same time, they try to plant seeds that will help others, never knowing when those seeds may take root. As one participant put it, "I understand that others have their own journey to untangle themselves from relying on animal products, and since I once was like them, I give them grace." Another stated, "I extend compassion toward others even when I don't agree with their choices. I live in alignment with my own morals and ethics, help anyone who asks me, and try to be an example so that people can see that plant-based living is approachable and doable."

The stories that follow illustrate the themes of nurturing vegan connections, along with courageous and empowered communication. First is the story of Stephanie Williams, the co-leader of Plant Based Capital Region, a whole-food, plant-based group in the Albany, New York, area that offers education, support, and fellowship for those interested in a plant-based lifestyle. During our interview, Stephanie shared the benefits of being part of a plant-based network, as well as her personal journey to become more confident in her communications with others.

Stephanie's story

Stephanie became vegetarian at age twenty, along with several friends, due to compassion for animals and concern about the environment. She noted that she took an environmental sociology class, which was "a big eye opener." At the time, she wasn't in touch with the health aspects of plant-based living, and "it was more around the environment and animal impacts."

She began dating Justin, who is now her husband, in 2019. He had been vegan for a couple of years. Stephanie said, "I decided to go vegan also because I'd been feeling called to move in that direction, but it had seemed too hard to do on my own." She indicated that they did not eat the healthiest vegan diet initially, relying heavily on eating out at restaurants as well as convenience foods. That year, Justin was diagnosed with Type 2 diabetes. He decided to try lifestyle changes, including a whole-food (vegan) diet, to see if he could reverse his diabetes without the need for medications. Stephanie joined him in this lifestyle change.

Justin had heard about a short-term "potato fast" as a way to reset taste buds and break free of entrenched eating patterns, including the addiction to foods high in sugar, salt, and fats. Stephanie and Justin did this reset for two weeks, then transitioned to a whole-food, plant-based lifestyle, free of processed foods as well as added salt, sugar, or oils. Stephanie said:

> The potato fast was hard, but it really helped to detox our bodies. I will also say it gave me a lot of information about my relationship with food, and what food meant to me emotionally. Going through it together also connected us as a couple. It was an emotional detox and awakening as well as a physical detox. Then we started whole-food plant-based living in January 2020. And we have never looked back.
>
> After shifting to eating whole plant foods, we both lost weight. After three months, my husband went to the doctor and his diabetes was gone. We started having more energy. Food tasted much better. Our bodies just started feeling healthier. Over the next several months, I also felt happier. Within nine months to a year, with my doctor's guidance, I was able to decrease the medications I had been taking for depression and anxiety. I was more present and less anxious.

Stephanie emphasized that her entire lifestyle was essential to healing emotionally and physically:

Although this diet and this way of eating has done so much for my mental health on its own, the whole lifestyle medicine approach was very important for me. I need stress management, I need to exercise, I need sleep. However, if I weren't eating healthy foods, the other stuff would not have the impact that it's having. Before I changed my diet, these other practices didn't have the impact that they have now in keeping me mentally and emotionally healthy.

When asked what her typical meals look like, she said,

In the morning, we eat a simple breakfast, like greens, fruit, seeds, and oatmeal, and for lunch, smoothies or salads, and then for dinner we usually find a recipe from a plant-based cooking show or the Forks Over Knives website or something like that. We try to incorporate Dr. Michael Greger's Daily Dozen[21] recommendations as much as possible. The focus on nutrients has been new for me and really helpful. I try to make it into a game where I put as many nutrients as possible into one meal. I've made it a challenge and we're always trying to find new ways to be creative, getting as many nutrients as possible.

She added,

We do still eat a lot of desserts. So that's my one battle—not eating too many desserts. That's been my battle for my whole life, even with whole-food, plant-based desserts. For sweeteners, we use dates, date sugar, or date paste, or occasionally raisins. I find that if I use other sweeteners, it affects my brain. I get a sugar high and then crash.

Stephanie noted that connecting with others who share her commitment to veganism and to whole-food nutrition has been one of the most meaningful parts of her journey. She indicated that soon after she and Justin adopted a whole-food vegan diet, they found a supportive plant-based community and were asked to become moderators. Soon after this, they met the leader of their local Plant Based Capital Region group, who needed help running the group. In time, Stephanie and Justin took over as co-leaders of the group. She noted that these experiences have been very fulfilling and have fueled her own commitment to a healthy lifestyle.

We've developed connections to a few different plant-based communities that have helped us along the way. It's great getting together with people who share the same values, to learn from each other, share resources, and ask questions. Even just going to a dinner or a potluck where you can eat everything on the table without having to give it a second thought, that is such a beautiful thing. For someone like me who loves food, shared meals give nurturance and community. Being able to fully participate in a meal, enjoying the food and nurturing people with the food I contribute has been lovely. I also love working together with others to impact things. That's always felt like part of my purpose, having a positive impact.

Stephanie acknowledged that social events with non-vegan friends and family have not always been easy, but she is developing skills to handle these situations more gracefully. She explained:

I have a lot of codependency. For a codependent people-pleaser, having to be in a group of people and take care of myself by eating differently than others is one of the hardest things. I feel like I've gotten much better, but I initially felt like a freak on a regular basis. I go on a retreat every year with this group of friends, and we all cook for each other. I didn't want to be a bother, I just wanted to say, "I'll cook everything for myself," but that's not how this group works. It's a supportive group of women and part of the experience is cooking for each other. I had to be okay with telling them my dietary needs and trust them to meet these needs. That's been really difficult. We've been doing this retreat since 2020 and this is the first year that I didn't feel bad about it the whole time. They have given me feedback that they feel good eating this way, like they are really nourishing their mind, body, and spirit on our retreat. These friends are truly a gift.

My family does not choose to accommodate my way of eating, because it's too much for them, so we bring our own food to family events. And that's okay for me. It works, because I understand that the way that my husband and I eat is such a departure from the way my family eats. It's been a challenge, but it's my family, and I can't not engage with them; I love them, and I want to be around them. Whereas in the past, maybe I would have chosen not to associate with people when there is so much difference in our beliefs. So, this has been a good challenge for me to learn from.

In the beginning, there was a lot of debate about who was right about things. I was very rigid, insisting that plant-based eating was the only way. And they would argue back that their way was the right way. It was really frustrating. My relationship with family has been helpful in learning how to meet people at the intersection of the things we do share. Which has helped me with carrying the message of plant-based living in a way that is relatable for other people. Because the truth is, I wholeheartedly believe in this way of life, but that doesn't mean I can convince others. However, I can show people the benefits. I think my life—the way I look, the way I feel, and my attitude—is a testament to how well this lifestyle works for me.

Stephanie's example highlights how she learned to include her own health and well-being in her circle of care, along with caring for other people, animals, and the planet. She is a role model for building community support and for discovering common ground that deepens connection, even among those who have different views and perspectives. She brings this passion for community and meaningful connection into a variety of roles: co-leading Plant Based Capital Region, assisting with Albany Veg Fest, and collaborating with a local animal sanctuary to create a retreat centered on principles of whole-food, plant-based living.

Deanna's story

Next is Deanna Meyler's story. She has a Ph.D. in sociology, is a Certified Master Vegan Lifestyle Coach and Educator, and currently works as director of development for a nonprofit clinic. At the time of our initial interview, she worked for the Peace Advocacy Network, an organization that provides education, support, and mentoring for a peaceful vegan lifestyle.

Deanna reported that her journey to a vegan lifestyle started with gastrointestinal issues when she was in high school. She stopped eating meat after her doctor advised her to avoid foods that were causing discomfort, which included animal protein. Eliminating meat helped to alleviate her GI discomfort. Several years later, she also eliminated dairy.

While in graduate school, she studied environmental sociology, with a focus on race, class, and gender issues. She said:

During this time, I learned about something called *window cows*,[22] which I had never heard of before. I was at an agricultural school.

I went to the place where these window cows were on campus, and I cried, it was awful. What they do is they cut a hole, about the size of my head, into the side of a cow, through the skin, the muscle, and bone, into their stomach. They put a rubber flap over it, so that the workers can actually reach their hands into the stomach of the cow and pull out the cud at any given moment. They leave it in indefinitely, I guess until the cow is no longer helpful to them.

And when I saw the cows with these windows in their sides, there was pus around it, lots of flies, and the cows had tears running down their faces. I didn't realize that cows have tears the way humans do. But I've since talked to people who run animal sanctuaries. They say that the only time they ever see cows with tears is when something very emotional happens to them. Like when a friend dies, or their baby cow is taken away, that kind of thing. So clearly, it's connected to their emotional state. These window cows looked awful, and their heads were bowed. They weren't eating, they were just bowed down. I cried. It was horrible. I realized I could no longer contribute to anything that was encouraging this kind of treatment to animals. At that point, I became fully vegan.

I later learned that this practice is fairly common for dairy cows. They take sterile dairy cows, and they put these windows in them. They do that because dairy cows are perpetually impregnated and being milked, so their microbiome is negatively impacted through that process. They use the window cows to pull the cud that has better microbiome health and give it to the dairy cows that are producing milk to help them do better. Without the dairy industry, we wouldn't need to do this. It slapped me in the face, and I realized, I have a choice not to support this.

Deanna indicated that initially she only knew one other vegan in her New Mexico, community, and there were few vegan options and products in the grocery store:

I ate a lot of rice and beans initially, and I taught myself how to cook. That ultimately led me to create a website, called *An Everyday Vegan*, that I've had now for over ten years. After I had been vegan for a while, a lot of people would come to me when they were ready to learn more. I kept answering the same handful of questions over and over again, so I finally decided to start a blog to respond to these questions. Then I attended Main Street Vegan Academy, and that's when I turned it into an actual website and started my coaching business thereafter.

She said, "Since becoming vegan, I have met amazing people. I've connected with some wonderful vegan friends. Even non-vegans, when they hear I am vegan, are usually understanding and supportive. Being vegan helps me recognize quickly which people are *not* supportive." Her husband was vegetarian when they first met. "We've been able to forge a life together where we are happy, with common goals and ideals and compassionate approaches to purchases and lifestyle and all these things. On our journey together, he was vegetarian, but vegan at home. He would have cheese pizza every now and then when he was out. However, he went vegan about a year ago."

When asked about her family's response to her veganism, Deanna said,

> They all knew I struggled with digesting animal proteins, so they were very tolerant of it. It doesn't necessarily mean they knew what to do with it, or that they were fully on board. But at least they would try to have vegan food for me at family gatherings and things like that.

Her work with the Peace Advocacy Network created meaningful vegan community in which she experienced connection, along with supporting and mentoring others. She said:

> I've always connected with social justice issues. Then I stumbled across the Peace Advocacy Network and got a job with them. And I'm so happy that I did. I feel very lucky to be able to spend all my work time on something that's so important to me. I get to meet all these amazing people who have the same ideals, and we're working towards a goal that we all believe in, that we feel is worth the time and the effort. I hope I can continue to help people make better choices for themselves. I run a vegan pledge program and help hundreds of people go vegan every year. I also wrote a big grant for funds to train people to be activists for the animals. I hope I can not only inspire people to go vegan, but also for them to take on the challenge to help others go vegan. Imagine the trickle down of that, imagine the power that can come from this empowerment happening in multiple communities, all over the world. That's a positive and exciting way for me to think about it. I'm starting here, I'm starting small, but hopefully, I can help it grow in a way that empowers, inspires, helps the animals as well as people.

In a subsequent conversation, Deanna noted that the grant for Peace Advocacy Network was ultimately funded, and she successfully built an activist training program to empower vegans to advocate and share their message more impactfully.

As highlighted through Stephanie's and Deanna's stories, and expressed throughout this chapter, meaningful connections are foundational and transformational. They can strengthen and reinforce our convictions, support us through challenges, bring us joy and fulfillment, and inspire us to be better versions of ourselves. We need relationships and communities that share our values, and we need skills to navigate our inevitable differences mindfully and effectively. Rather than seeing those who are different as "the enemy," we can find common ground in our shared humanity. Read on for suggestions to deepen your own experience of connection.

Action Steps

The following are reflection questions and actions to increase meaningful and supportive connections in your life:

- **Assess your current level of support.**
    - List the people in your life you can count on to listen and be there when you are going through a hard time or to celebrate with when good things happen.
    - Whom do you enjoy spending time with for fun and enjoyable activities?
    - Who supports and encourages you on your plant-based and/or vegan journey?
    - Whom do you turn to for guidance, information, and insights?
    - When you consider the preceding questions, are there areas of support that are lacking or missing in your life? What actions might you take to build more support?
- **Investigate vegan groups locally and/or online.** Explore and find a group, program, or network that resonates for you. Some groups focus more on the nutritional and health aspects of plant-based living, while others may focus on ethical issues, animal protection, and/

or the environment. Some groups or programs are geared toward helping people transition to a vegan lifestyle and provide resources and recipes to help. Some are local in-person groups, while others are virtual online networks. Do a search online or on social media to find vegan groups. In addition, there is a list of vegan organizations in this book's Resources section. Select a few that you want to explore.

- **Identify and reframe limiting beliefs that hold you back from satisfying connections with others.** Many of us have learned beliefs that hold us back from seeking support or connection, or from expressing our needs. If you are not fully satisfied with your relationships, see if any of these limiting messages (listed next) are interfering, and reframe them with more hopeful, empowering, and realistic messages that invite receptivity to support and connection.

    o   I'm weak if I need support.
        (*Reframe*: It is human to need support, and it brings me closer to others.)

    o   I need to figure things out on my own.
        (*Reframe*: _____)

    o   I don't want to be a bother or burden.
        (*Reframe*: _____)

    o   I don't want to be judged or seen as different.
        (*Reframe*: _____)

    o   If I receive support, I feel indebted.
        (*Reframe*: _____)

    o   I don't deserve support.
        (*Reframe*: _____)

    o   To be a good person, I need to give more than I receive.
        (*Reframe*: _____)

    o   Others don't want to know what I feel or need.
        (*Reframe*: _____)

    o   Others are insensitive or self-centered.
        (*Reframe*: _____)

    o   Others don't "get" me.
        (*Reframe*: _____)

As you reframe these old, limiting beliefs with more empowering messages, what insights do you have for how you might strengthen your relationships and support network?

- **Proactively prepare for challenges and enlist support.** What challenges do you have with others not understanding or supporting your values or lifestyle? List situations that cause difficulties for you (e.g., shared meals, social gatherings, holiday traditions, travel). If you are moving toward a vegan lifestyle, what social difficulties do you anticipate? Develop a plan for proactively speaking up with others who are involved. Let them know your commitment to a plant-based lifestyle, the changes you will be making, and what support you would like from them. Consider strengthening your communication skills by checking out some of the Resources for thriving emotionally and socially in the back of the book. In addition, we will delve deeper into strategies for improving communication and enlisting support in Chapters Nine and Ten.

Developing meaningful connections is one of the joys that can come with discovering your passions and sharing them with others, and for many it is a fulfilling aspect of their vegan journey. Along with healthy relationships, it is also important to become empowered on your own behalf. The next chapter shares how a nutritious vegan lifestyle can empower you to take charge of your health.

CHAPTER 7

TAKE CHARGE OF
YOUR HEALTH

"Let food be thy medicine and medicine thy food."

—**Hippocrates**

"The doctor of the future will give no medicine but will instruct
his patient in the care of [the] human frame in diet and in the
cause and prevention of diseases."

—**Thomas Edison**

Our health crisis

Chronic illness takes a huge toll. I have witnessed its impact on the lives
of many of my clients, my parents, and numerous friends and family.
For those afflicted with a chronic medical condition, it often takes a toll
on their very quality of life—impacting everything from daily activities,
to work, to relationships, to finances, to independence and autonomy.
Enjoyable activities may become much more difficult or even impossible.
Dreams for the future may be sidelined, as the focus shifts to healing,
and when that's not possible, simply sustaining and adjusting to the new
normal. Far too often, chronic disease diminishes full engagement in life,
as well as the duration of life.

Chronic medical conditions also create a huge societal toll. In the
United States, we are facing a large-scale health crisis. It affects our
country's economic well-being, as disability takes workers out of the
workforce, and we spend huge amounts on medical care. In fact, the
United States spends more per capita on healthcare than any other
nation. Healthcare expenditures totaled $4.5 trillion in 2022, which comes
out to $13,493 per person.[1] Healthcare costs in the United States are

double those of other countries with comparable socioeconomic status, including Australia, Canada, Japan, and Western European countries.[2] Despite the United State's high healthcare spending, its residents have lower life expectancy than those in other high-income nations.[3] While the COVID-19 pandemic greatly increased healthcare costs in 2020, these trends toward rising medical expenditures have been going on for decades and are anticipated to further accelerate in future years.

According to the Centers for Disease Control and Prevention (CDC), 90 percent of our healthcare costs are directed toward treating and managing chronic medical conditions, including heart disease, stroke, Type 2 diabetes, arthritis, Alzheimer's disease, epilepsy, dental disease, and mental health disorders.[4] Some of these chronic conditions are among the top causes of death in the United States, with cardiovascular disease leading the way. The CDC reported that there were 695,547 deaths due to heart disease in 2021, followed next by cancer (605,213 deaths) and COVID-19 (416,893 deaths). Stroke, respiratory diseases, Alzheimer's disease, and diabetes were also among the leading causes of death.[5]

Cardiovascular disease in particular has become epidemic in the United States. Drawing on data from the American Heart Association, AARP reports that over 75 percent of people between ages sixty and seventy-nine, and 90 percent of those over age eighty, are afflicted with some form of cardiovascular disease.[6] Additionally, research suggests that heart disease often starts when we are young, long before we see any signs of its progression. Autopsies of three hundred male US soldiers who died during the Korean War (at an average age of twenty-two years) found visible evidence of heart disease in over three-quarters of the soldiers, even though they had never been diagnosed with any cardiovascular problems.[7]

Infectious diseases were the top causes of death in the early 1900's; today, the leading causes are predominantly degenerative lifestyle-related diseases. These are what Dr. T. Colin Campbell, the author of *The China Study*, calls "diseases of affluence."[8] There are likely multiple factors that contributed to this shift. Improved sanitation and medications such as antibiotics have lessened certain infectious diseases. However, it is not just that we are living longer, and therefore having more degenerative diseases. Dr. Michael Greger, author of *How Not to Die*, explains that the onslaught of chronic disease has been strongly associated with a shift in our dietary patterns. With the industrial revolution and other cultural changes, most Western cultures now eat a diet dominated by animal-based and highly processed foods.[9]

Those in affluent countries generally eat ample calories, but many of these calories come from unhealthy foods. On average, Americans get only 11 percent of their calories from plant foods (e.g., fruits, vegetables, legumes, nuts, and whole grains), and about half of these calories come from less healthy plant-based foods, such as french fries, potato chips, ketchup, and apple pie. Most of Americans' calories come from animal foods, such as meat, dairy, eggs, and fish (33 percent), and processed foods, including baked goods, refined grains, sodas, sweets, and other products with added salt, oils, and/or sugar (56 percent).[10]

The power of plants

Interestingly, as shown by research in the Blue Zones, those living in geographic locations that consume more whole plant foods have lower rates of these chronic degenerative diseases. They tend to live longer, while enjoying healthier, more active, and vibrant lives.[11] Unfortunately, as more and more developing countries shift to a Western diet, with increased processed food, fast food, and animal-sourced foods, they are also experiencing increases in lifestyle-related chronic diseases, such as diabetes, heart disease, and stroke.[12] In addition, those who emigrate to the United States from countries with low rates of degenerative disease tend to experience increased risk of chronic disease upon moving there and adopting the Western diet.[13]

The China Study highlights the strong relationship between diet and risk of chronic and degenerative disease. Co-authored by Dr. T. Colin Campbell and his son Thomas M. Campbell, it shares years of comprehensive research in a clear and understandable way. This research includes Dr. Campbell's laboratory studies, which found that consumption of animal protein (but not plant protein) stimulated the initiation, promotion, and progression of cancer in rats. It also covers the research that gave the book its title, a large-scale epidemiological study in China, examining relationships between dietary patterns and disease. The China Study, led by Dr. Campbell and colleagues from Cornell University, Oxford University, and the Chinese Academy of Preventive Medicine, is hailed as one of the largest and most comprehensive epidemiological studies ever conducted. The *New York Times* called the China Study "the Grand Prix of epidemiology." This research found that higher consumption of plant foods, along with the fiber and antioxidants they contain, was associated with lower blood cholesterol and lower rates of cancer and heart disease, compared to diets higher in animal foods.[14]

The China Study book is fascinating, and a must-read for anyone who wants to understand the links between diet, nutrition, and health. In addition to sharing Dr. Campbell's research, it comprehensively reviews the vast research literature on diet and disease, showing that there is ample existing evidence for the benefits of a whole-food, plant-based diet in reducing risk of many chronic and degenerative diseases. The book also sheds light on the political and economic factors that play into why most of us don't even know about these research findings.

Once you delve into the vast research evidence showing the benefits of a plant-powered diet for human health, you might wonder why you haven't learned about this before. Most often, we are steered toward medications and procedures as the only solutions for managing disease, and we aren't even told about the power of nutrition and lifestyle changes for preventing and reversing disease, or given guidance for how to implement them. Perhaps the substantially higher reimbursement rates for pharmaceuticals and surgeries compared to lifestyle or nutritional counseling plays a part in this. When nutrition is mentioned at all, the information is often confusing or conflicting, based on the latest fad, opinion, or preference, and steeped in our society's proclivity for an animal-based diet.[15] When I read *The China Study* and other research on plant-based nutrition, I wondered, "Why don't we all know this?" It seems so obvious, but it's as if we have blinders. And of course, there are many corporate interests whose economic well-being depends on us not knowing.

How simple it is, and yet so hard, for us to see the healing that happens when we return to nature, and enjoy the foods that come from the bounty of the earth. As highlighted in previous chapters, plant-based nutrition gives us fiber, micronutrients, and antioxidants that help our body fight disease and inflammation. A high-nutrient plant-sourced diet strengthens our immune system, gives us energy and vitality, helps us maintain a healthy weight, strengthens our mental and cognitive health, and, in many cases, can heal or reverse disease.

Plant-based pioneers

The research on the health benefits of a plant-based diet is so vast, I don't have the space to cover it in all the depth it deserves. However, I will give an overview of the work of some leading plant-based doctors to showcase the power of plant-based nutrition for better health:

- **Dr. Dean Ornish**, whom I referenced in Chapter Six, conducted revolutionary research showing that a healthy lifestyle, centered around a plant-based diet, stress management, exercise, and group support, can reverse coronary artery disease, even among those with advanced cases. In addition to improvements in patients' physical symptoms, functioning, and well-being, scans of their blood vessels showed reduced blockage and improved blood flow. Dr. Ornish has found similar results with men who had early-stage prostate cancer, halting the progression of cancer when they followed his plant-based lifestyle program. And in collaboration with Nobel Prize winner Dr. Elizabeth Blackburn, he found that after three months on his plant-based lifestyle program, participants increased the length of their telomeres. Telomeres are the ends of chromosomes that regulate aging. Generally, our telomeres shorten as we age, and this process can be accelerated by stress and other lifestyle factors. Shorter telomeres are associated with increased risk of premature death from degenerative disease. However, Drs. Ornish and Blackburn found that patients who made healthy lifestyle changes evidenced lengthening of telomeres while control subjects had a decrease in telomere length over time. Greater adherence to a healthy lifestyle was associated with greater telomere growth.[16] Dr. Ornish has written several books and is featured in documentaries including *The Game Changers* and *Eating You Alive*.

- **Dr. Caldwell Esselstyn, Jr.** began research in the 1980s examining the effects of a whole-food, plant-based diet for patients with severe cardiovascular disease. He found that patients who followed a low-fat, plant-based diet showed significant reductions in total cholesterol, LDL cholesterol, and coronary events and symptoms, while regaining their functioning and quality of life. Many showed visible reductions in blockages in their arteries. Dr. Esselstyn wrote the book *Prevent and Reverse Heart Disease*[17] and is featured in the documentary *Forks Over Knives*.

- **Dr. Joel Fuhrman** has become well-known through sharing his work in various PBS specials on nutrition. He guides patients to adopt a nutrient-dense, plant-based diet, which he calls a Nutritarian diet. Dr. Fuhrman uses the acronym G-BOMBS as a handy reminder of the high-nutrient foods he recommends consuming regularly: Greens, Beans, Onions, Mushrooms, Berries, and Seeds.[18] Dr. Fuhrman has written several books, including *Eat for Life*,[19] and is a regular speaker at plant-based health and nutrition conferences.

- **Dr. Neal Barnard** is the president of the Physicians Committee for Responsible Medicine (PCRM), which advocates a healthy plant-based diet, and hosts a twenty-one-day Vegan Kickstart to help people transition to a plant-based lifestyle. PCRM is also a strong proponent for ethical and effective medical research models that don't involve the use or harm of animals. Barnard has pioneered research showing the benefits of plant-based nutrition in reversing Type 2 diabetes,[20] as well as reducing hormonal and menopause symptoms.[21] He has written numerous books, including *The Cheese Trap* and *Power Foods for the Brain*.[22]

- **Dr. Brooke Goldner** was diagnosed with an aggressive form of lupus, an autoimmune disease that attacks the body's tissues and/or organs, when she was only 16 years old. After extensive medical treatment, she was able to attain remission, but dealt with side effects and physical limitations. She maintained remission during college, but during the stress of attending medical school, had a severe flare-up, along with the onset of blood clots. She underwent medication therapies that helped her symptoms but had serious side effects. As expressed by Dr. Goldner in her book, *Goodbye Lupus*, "Once again, modern medicine had saved my life, but it was not giving me health."[23] It was when she was trying to lose weight for her wedding, through the help of her fiancé (who is an expert in fitness and metabolism), that she discovered the healing power of a whole-food, plant-based diet. Within a few months on this eating plan, she not only lost weight, but felt much better physically. She no longer had aches and pains and had increased energy. When she had bloodwork, she found that she had no signs of lupus, and has remained healthy and free of disease ever since. After completing her medical training, she developed programs to help others who suffer from autoimmune disease, teaching them how to adopt the same whole-food, high-raw, plant-based protocol that helped her to heal. You can learn more about Dr. Goldner's story and her healing protocol through her books *Goodbye Lupus* and *Goodbye Autoimmune Disease*.[24]

- **Dr. Kristi Funk** is a board-certified breast cancer surgeon and best-selling author of the book, *Breasts: The Owner's Manual*. She discovered the scientific evidence for the health benefits of a whole-food, plant-based (WFPB) diet while writing her book. She acknowledged that prior to diving into this research, she was convinced that her diet of chicken, turkey, fish, and vegetables was healthy, but upon reading the science, she and her family adopted a WFPB diet, and she now encourages her patients to eat this way as well. She admits that she was surprised to learn the benefits of whole or minimally processed soy (e.g., edamame, tofu, tempeh, soybeans, and soy milk) for breast health. She discovered that rather than increasing hormonal estrogen as many people fear, the isoflavones in soy actually block the estrogen receptors that fuel cancer growth. She is a proponent for integrating lifestyle approaches, along with standard medical and surgical care when they are needed.[25]

- **Drs. Dean and Ayesha Sherzai** are co-directors of the Alzheimer's Prevention Program at Loma Linda University Medical Center. They have created a lifestyle program for cognitive and neurological health that includes plant-based nutrition, exercise, stress management, adequate rest and sleep, and cognitive activities to challenge the brain. They assert, based on their research and clinical findings, that 90 percent of Alzheimer's cases can be prevented with these healthy nutrition and lifestyle practices, and the remaining 10 percent who have strong genetic risk can potentially delay the onset by ten to fifteen years. They are authors of *The Alzheimer's Solution*, which describes their comprehensive program for preventing and reversing cognitive decline.[26]

- **Dr. Michael Greger** is an internationally recognized speaker on nutrition and public health issues. His presentations are down-to-earth and engaging, bringing humor while sharing the vast research on diet and health in understandable and accessible ways. He authored the books *How Not to Die*, *How Not to Diet*, and *How Not to Age*. His nonprofit website, NutritionFacts.org, is an extremely helpful resource, providing a wealth of articles and videos covering the latest nutrition research.[27]

There are numerous other physicians and researchers who have been foundational in raising awareness of the health benefits of plant-powered nutrition, including Dr. Milton Mills, Dr. Michael Klaper, Dr. John McDougall, Dr. Will Bulsiewicz, Dr. Saray Stancic, and Dr. Joel Kahn, to name just a few. In the Resources section at the back of this book, I have included a list of books, websites, documentaries, and other media to explore if you'd like to learn more.

Take back your power

While the research on the healing power of a plant-based diet is, in and of itself, incredibly inspiring, what I find even more uplifting is the discovery that we have more power over our health than we've been taught to believe. When we take charge of our health, it affects not only our physical well-being, but also our sense of agency and emotional well-being. During the first several years of my clinical psychology training and career, I specialized in health and medical psychology, working with patients who had chronic medical conditions and/or chronic pain. I witnessed the interplay between psychological and physical health in dealing with these chronic conditions. On the one hand, chronic illness has a negative emotional impact when it robs people of their ability to engage in enjoyable activities, and disrupts relationships, work, and daily self-care. And, on the other hand, patients' emotional state and mindset influences how they handle their medical problems. I saw that those who felt some degree of empowerment were more likely to heal, and even if they didn't fully recover, they were able to experience greater quality of life and engagement in meaningful activities.

Early in my career, I learned about the power of our thinking styles, mindset, stress management, exercise, and other lifestyle factors for influencing health, but I had little understanding of the role of nutrition. When I became vegetarian and first learned about the research shared in this chapter, I was blown away. I hadn't realized the degree to which our diet and lifestyle can influence our health. Learning that we aren't entirely at the mercy of genes, circumstances, or the medical system, and that we can take charge of our own health, was eye-opening and empowering. I wanted to share this epiphany with others.

I witnessed both of my parents go through lifestyle-related illnesses. My mother died from lung cancer at only sixty-two years old. My father, who dealt with surgeries and complications from cardiovascular disease for the last decade of his life, died at age seventy-four. In both cases, I longed to share information with them or do something to change the outcome. When my mother was diagnosed with cancer, I gave her the book, *Love, Medicine, and Miracles* by Bernie Siegel, perhaps hoping that its wisdom would lead to some kind of miracle in halting her cancer. After my father went through bypass surgery, I sent a copy of Dean Ornish's cookbook, wanting to share the healing potential of lifestyle change. (I don't think he ever tried the recipes, but he seemed to appreciate my positive intentions.) However, their medical conditions progressed, and ultimately, I had to accept that I was powerless to change this. I was heartbroken to witness how their illnesses savaged their lives and their dreams. My grief was compounded by their passing at a younger age than I anticipated. Even though I was an adult when I lost them, I felt very much like an orphan after their deaths.

I believe the loss of my parents played a role in my own desire to be as proactive as possible with my own health, so that I can remain independent, vibrant, and healthy for as long as possible. I have experienced firsthand the sense of empowerment that can come with taking charge of my diet and lifestyle. For me, it started with a commitment to exercise. I have always been fairly active, but in my thirties, I began regular strength training, as well as cardio. I also integrated other forms of self-care, such as meditation, journaling, and spiritual practices. Shortly before I became vegetarian, I started to move away from my unhealthy patterns of daily sweets and microwave meals, to at least do a little cooking and bring healthier snacks to work. When I had my awakening to become vegetarian (and later, vegan) I read up on the nutritional aspects of a plant-based diet and learned how to maximize my nutrition, to do my best to get all the nutrients I needed. I began cooking regularly and eating many more fruits and veggies than ever before.

I have seen the healing power of plants in my own life. Since eating plant-based, I have maintained a healthy weight, had fewer colds and illnesses, and enjoyed greater energy. Unlike many people my age, I don't take any medications other than vitamins. When I gave up dairy, I eliminated seasonal allergy symptoms and gained clearer skin. And beyond that, it feels great to actively manage my own well-being, to be empowered, rather than heavily relying on the medical or pharmaceutical industries. I am grateful for the help of traditional medical care, that it is there when I or others truly need it. However, I have come to realize that we have significantly more personal power over our health than many of us realize. Rather than clogging our arteries with the Standard American Diet (SAD), we can make healthy dietary choices that improve our well-being and decrease our risk for degenerative lifestyle diseases.

Wanda Huberman, executive director of the National Health Association (referenced in Chapter Four), is an inspiring example of taking back her power through a healthy plant-based lifestyle. She said,

> [Since becoming plant-based], I maintain a healthy weight. I have no medical concerns. I wake up with energy and gratitude every day. I have mental clarity and focus that allows me to accomplish most of what I set out to do on a daily basis. I have the strength to do daily

workouts and energy to play with my grandchildren. I strive to take responsibility for my health and want to do what I can to live a long healthy life full of vitality and independence.

Many of the vegans I surveyed shared this sense of health empowerment, as illustrated in the survey responses here:

"I feel free, empowered to take charge of my own health."

"After over a decade of medication and many different prescriptions over that period, I was liberated. I have regained clarity, purpose, humanity, intelligence and so much more. Life is meaningful and amazing. I have regained life and hope. Day by day, everything keeps improving."

"I have a healthier relationship with food, treat my body better, and feel more comfortable with my body."

"In stressful times, I remind myself of the power of plants to heal me and make me a ready warrior for the things that life will bring. This gives me a sense of peace. I now have a stronger immune system, a way to age without medication, and so much more energy and clarity. I am grateful for all the precious little things."

"I enjoy what I eat and feel very connected to my food, knowing that my body temple is receiving the best nourishment and love it can get."

"I feel more in control of my life because I have accurate knowledge of how to take care of my body, and I no longer feel as confused or manipulated by false advertisement, misinformation, or food lobbying."

Eat whole plant foods

To optimize the benefits of a vegan diet, eat plenty of *whole* plant foods. This means plants that are as close to their original state as possible, either unprocessed or minimally processed. Many years ago, being vegan meant eating mostly whole plant foods because there weren't a lot of vegan processed foods available. Now we are blessed with an abundance of commercial vegan products, including plant-based cheeses, milks, sour creams, ice cream, meat substitutes, pizzas, and baked goods. These options are delicious, add flavor and texture to meals, and make life easier, so we don't always have to cook from scratch. Vegan convenience foods are especially helpful when transitioning to a vegan lifestyle. However, the research suggests that over-reliance on processed foods (especially those that are ultra-processed, with extra-long ingredient lists, additives, and excessive sugar, oil, and/or salt) does not bring optimal health,[28] so it is best to get most of your calories from whole foods and enjoy processed foods as an occasional treat.[29] [30]

What do I mean by whole plant foods? This includes all kinds of leafy greens, cruciferous vegetables like broccoli and cauliflower, colorful veggies of all kinds, fruits, mushrooms, beans, lentils, nuts, seeds, and whole grains like brown rice, quinoa, millet, oats, and farro. In addition, research and clinical findings suggest that including lots of *raw* fruits and veggies boosts health, immunity, and vitality. For example, Dr. Brooke Goldner, whom I mentioned earlier, has helped numerous patients regain their health from severe autoimmune disease through a high-raw whole-food vegan diet.

Responses from my vegan research participants highlighted the benefits of eating whole plant foods. Slightly over half of the survey respondents reported that they ate a whole-food, plant-based (WFPB) vegan diet, limiting highly processed foods and, in many cases, oils, sugar, and salt. Some of these WFPB vegans reported strict avoidance of processed foods, while others reported consuming occasional vegan convenience foods and commercially made treats. Most of the remaining survey participants (over 40 percent) reported no particular diet philosophy beyond eating vegan (e.g., "I don't worry about what I eat, as long as there are no animal products in it.")

Many participants who ate predominantly WFPB commented that they felt much better health-wise when they consumed whole plant foods and avoided highly processed foods, especially those high in oils and sugar. This comment by one participant reflects the experience shared by several: "It still amazes me at how great I feel when I eat WFPB rather than processed foods. I've tried many diets before, and I still felt bad. WFPB is the key to feeling great all over. When I eat healthier, I feel fantastic the day after; I'm not achy and have so much more energy. I'm sure that dairy and meat only compounded this effect before I went vegan."

Lifestyle Medicine

More physicians and healthcare providers are recognizing the importance of nutrition and lifestyle for improving health. In response to this growing movement, the American College of Lifestyle Medicine (ACLM) was founded in 2004.[31] The ACLM is a professional medical society for physicians and other providers that offers training and certification in evidence-based lifestyle approaches. Lifestyle medicine is a whole-person approach and focuses on preventing, treating, and reversing chronic disease. Healthcare providers using this approach are guided by six pillars:

1. A whole-food, plant-predominant diet
2. Consistent physical activity
3. Stress management
4. Restorative sleep
5. Social connections
6. Avoidance of harmful substances

Vegan fitness

Not only can a whole-food, vegan diet prevent and heal many diseases, but it can also take you to your next level of fitness. Many people have the idea that they need meat to get enough protein and thrive as an athlete. However, the prowess of numerous vegan athletes and fitness enthusiasts shows otherwise. Plant-based athletes discover that plant nutrition more than adequately fuels their workouts, as well as increases one's strength, decreases the risk of injury, and enhances post-workout recovery. Here are some plant-powered athletes who have excelled in their sport: Venus Williams (tennis legend), Derrick Morgan (football), Carl Lewis (Olympic track and field), Meagan Duhamel (Olympic figure skater), Scott Jurek (ultramarathoner), Dotsie Bausch (Olympic cyclist), and Rich Roll (ultra-endurance athlete).

To learn more about vegan fitness and athletics, consider watching the engaging and informative documentary, *The Game Changers*,[32] which shares athletes' stories as well as the science behind plant-powered nutrition.

Another great resource is the book, *The Plant-Based Athlete* authored by Matt Frazier (ultrarunner and host of the *No Meat Athlete* podcast) and Robert Cheeke (natural body-building champion and author of *Shred It*).[33] In addition, several vegan athletes have written memoirs sharing their journeys and their wisdom as plant-based athletes. For example, *Finding Ultra* shares Rich Roll's inspiring story of moving from addiction and poor health to becoming an ultra-endurance athlete in his forties, as well as his tips for a healthy plant-fueled lifestyle.[34]

The fitness benefits of a vegan lifestyle were exemplified by some of the vegans I interviewed. For example, Geoff Palmer, age sixty at the time of our interview, has been vegan for over thirty-five years and is a Natural Bodybuilding and Natural Physique Masters champion. ("Natural" bodybuilders do not use steroids or other drugs to build muscle.) He is founder and CEO of Clean Machine, a plant-based fitness nutrition company, and organized the world's first all-vegan natural bodybuilding competition, the World Vegan Bodybuilding Championship. Geoff's intense workouts at the gym and his muscled physique (while wearing a vegan T-shirt) inspire others to realize that you can indeed be fit and strong with a healthy, plant-based diet.

Angela Fischetti, founder of Boomer and Beyond Wellness, is a fitness and yoga instructor as well as a massage therapist who specializes in working with older adults. She embodies a passion for fitness and healthy living, which she shares with her clients. Angela, who previously struggled with serious medical issues, an eating disorder, and emotional issues, claimed her best health (and mental health) when she adopted a super-clean whole-food, plant-based diet. She follows the *SOFAS-free* approach taught by plant-based culinary guru Chef AJ, eating an abundance of whole plant foods while avoiding added Sugar, Oil, Flour, Alcohol, and Salt.[35] With this lifestyle, she has experienced greater emotional well-being and improved her health, strength, fitness, and endurance.

Many vegans discover similar health empowerment, as well as improved vitality and fitness, when they adopt a whole-food vegan lifestyle. The following are the stories of Jeniece, Linda, Sally, Nivi, and Bob and Fran, who each took charge of their health through plant-powered living.

Jeniece's story

Jeniece Paige runs Black Vegan Health and Wellness Coaching and is a doctoral student in holistic health and nutrition. Her journey to becoming vegan started in 1990. She said:

> I was sick; I was just recovering from a tubal pregnancy that nearly took my life. I was overweight, I didn't feel good. I didn't like the way I saw myself. My mom was just diagnosed with high blood pressure. My grandmother also had high blood pressure and was starting to have some related problems, like strokes and heart issues. So, I saw these health problems in my family, and after the experience I had with my tubal pregnancy, I knew I needed to do something. I decided to become vegetarian. It was a weight loss journey for me at first—knowing that with my family history and being overweight, I was well on my way to having health problems. I gave up dairy, red meat, and pork. I did not have a clue what I was doing, and I didn't know about the different levels of a vegetarian lifestyle. I didn't go all the way, because at that time, doctors thought animal protein was best. So, I just had chicken, one breast a week, and nothing else.
>
> What transformed me is I started going to the half-price bookstore, found vegetarian books and cookbooks, and learned vegetarian cooking. I started self-educating. That's how I learned about veganism. I wanted to be vegan, but my doctor was telling me I needed animal protein so my body could heal. And then one week when we were traveling, I went to KFC to have my one piece of chicken and ended up with food poisoning. That was for the best, because I was able to walk away from having that weekly chicken breast and become a vegan.
>
> When I transitioned to a vegan lifestyle, my health started to get better. I learned how to cook and the benefits of using herbs and spices. I started losing weight and felt amazing. My skin cleared up. Just from feeding my body properly and educating myself at the same time. I also got stronger and able to exercise better.
>
> Over time, people started noticing my transition. They saw me lose weight and get fit; they asked me what I was doing, and could I help them? That's how my coaching came about. I went on to get a personal training certification. I also have my master's in business and am currently working on a Ph.D. in holistic nutrition. I help women with hormonal issues, healthy weight loss, and gut health, so they can move away from yo-yo dieting and create sustainable health and wellness practices.

Linda's story

Linda Middlesworth is the founder of VeganMentor Health Coaching. In addition, she is a nutrition and cooking instructor for Physicians Committee for Responsible Medicine (PCRM), event planner for Get Healthy Live, and organizer of the Sacramento Vegan Society. Her story is a testament to the healing power of a whole-food vegan lifestyle for reversing health conditions, achieving and maintaining a healthy weight, and vibrant and beautiful aging. She was seventy-eight years old at the time of our interview, and still teaching aerobics and personal training at her gym. Linda's vegan journey started over thirty years ago, when she was in her mid-forties. She explained:

> I had heart disease, thyroid cancer, and was fifty pounds overweight. I had prediabetes, high blood pressure, and elevated cholesterol. I was very sick. My neighbor told me about Dr. John McDougall. I went out and bought his book (*The McDougall Program: 12 Days to Dynamic Health*) and read it from cover to cover. It showed all these people who had changed their diet to a plant-exclusive, oil-free diet, and recovered from problems like coronary heart disease and diabetes. I started following the guidance from his book. I wasn't perfect. At first, I still had red wine every evening. And I ate french fries because I was so addicted to them. But overall, I followed Dr. McDougall's program, and I started to lose weight. I wasn't losing weight as quickly as I'd like, so I decided to get very clean with my eating. I really followed the program, and that's when I took off all the extra weight that I didn't want anymore. I never felt better in my life.
>
> I realized that all the things I had learned before about health and diet were wrong. I didn't know that a plant-based diet could reverse things like Type 2 diabetes. I had prediabetes, but my doctors didn't tell me to change to a high-starch plant diet. No, it was nothing like that. They said my food was fine, that it wasn't my food, I was just an unlucky lady. I know they meant well; they didn't know about any of this either.
>
> After changing to a whole-food, plant-based diet, I started feeling on top of the world. Within a short time, I lost fifty pounds, my cholesterol and blood pressure improved, and I was no longer prediabetic. My cancer even went into remission. I felt light on my feet for the first time. I was an aerobics instructor, and I could jump

higher and be more active and a better example to my aerobics students and personal training clients. At the time, I was also a graphic designer, and felt more confident when I met new clients because I looked and felt better.

Later on, I learned what happened to dairy cows and other farm animals, and I became an ethical vegan as well. I started to feel good because I was not killing any creatures anymore. I love food, and I was so happy to know that I could live without hurting anybody. I've been a big animal lover all my life. My mental health really went up after that. Then I started holding plant-based groups, where I met more people like me, and I wasn't alone anymore.

I didn't know what my purpose was before. But the moment I found out about the gulags of despair that farm animals live in—that's when I knew I had to help. I started the Sacramento Vegan Society, which now has over 5,000 members. I'm also a Food For Life instructor with Dr. Neal Barnard and run my VeganMentor health coaching program to help people move toward a healthy, plant-powered lifestyle.

Sally's story

Sally Lipsky, Ph.D., is a retired professor of education and leads Plant-Based Pittsburgh, a nonprofit organization whose mission is to educate and support community members trying to adopt healthy plant-based eating patterns. She authored the book *Beyond Cancer: The Powerful Effect of Plant-Based Eating*. She practices meditation and is a yoga instructor. Her journey to a whole-food, plant-exclusive lifestyle started after her diagnosis with cancer. She explained:

> I had a startling diagnosis of late-stage ovarian cancer in 2007. Because the symptoms are so subtle, ovarian cancer is often diagnosed at an advanced stage. I immediately had surgery and months of chemotherapy. After chemotherapy, there was no sign of cancer, but I was ever-vigilant because I learned that people with this late-stage diagnosis often have cancer return within two years. I was always extremely anxious before my blood work and scans, wondering when it would come back. Then I happened to read an article in the local paper about Dr. David Servan-Schreiber, a neuroscientist who had brain cancer and wrote a book called

Anti-Cancer: A New Way of Life. In his interview, he talked about the relationship between food and lifestyle and cancer. This opened my eyes, and I started researching more.

Before my diagnosis, I thought I was healthy. I was a middle-aged woman who followed all the guidelines to care for my health. I exercised regularly and ate lean animal protein (chicken) along with dairy and eggs. I had no idea about the connection between food and disease. After reading that article, I started to attend the Vegan Summerfest and went to conferences, where I discovered the benefits of a whole-food, plant-based lifestyle. I also learned about the Blue Zones. I didn't get this information easily; I had to dig for it. My background as an education professor led me to research and learn more, and later to want to teach others.

Dairy was the last thing to go, because we're told we need it for strong bones. But by 2009, I was fully plant-based. The key thing that I gained from being plant-based was a sense of empowerment. I also started practicing yoga regularly, which helped settle my mind and body. I've gotten to the point where cancer isn't as scary to me now as it was fourteen years ago, because there is some control. I have not had a recurrence of cancer. This way of living has been a lifesaver. My energy increased, and there's an overall feeling of well-being. Nothing is a cure-all, but this lifestyle has helped me stay cancer-free.

Nivi's story

Coming from a background in international brand strategy and marketing, Nivi Jaswal-Wirtjes pivoted her career trajectory after healing through a whole-food, plant-based diet. She subsequently founded the Virsa Foundation and the JIVINITI research and advocacy program to raise awareness around plant-based nutrition, public health, and planetary health, with a focus on reaching nutritionally underserved populations. In addition to holding a BA in psychology and an MBA, Nivi is a board-certified health and wellness coach. She is also a certified Lifestyle Medicine coach and Jungian coach.

At age thirty-four, in 2015, Nivi received some unexpected clinical diagnoses. She discovered she had prediabetes, polycystic ovarian syndrome, hypothyroidism, premenstrual dysphoric disorder, severe edema, metabolic syndrome, and insulin resistance. She also experienced severe, chronic insomnia. Her doctors gave her a grim prognosis, saying that she would need to be on hormone replacement therapy for the rest of her life. She was also told that she would likely need a hysterectomy in the future. After learning of her diagnoses, she was deeply distressed:

> It was horrible. I took a long walk afterward. I was reflecting, thinking, "Where did life go wrong?" I thought I was successful in the corporate world, but suddenly it dawned on me that if I weren't healthy, all the success, money, and wealth that I was accumulating wouldn't mean much. At the time of my diagnosis, I was on a keto diet, which had been recommended by a sports endocrinologist at a prestigious hospital. I thought that I was relatively healthy, and that all the things that were happening to me were par for the course due to genetics. Certain diseases were present in my family, and I thought I could only delay them, not prevent them. I thought of them as a genetic infection I could only try to run away from, and that it would eventually catch up to me—but not this soon!
>
> A few months after my diagnoses, I met with a nutritionist who was a proponent of plant-based diets, and I remember arguing with her. I was angry that she was questioning my protein paradigm. I felt like she didn't get me or the personal genetic context I was coming from. I had lost all my grandparents to chronic illness by the time I turned eighteen. My dad had been diagnosed with Type 2 diabetes, and I saw him go from a sociable, happy person to one who was cognitively high functioning, but emotionally depressed. I believed that the only way to delay these health issues for myself was to follow a high-protein, animal-centric diet. I paid very little heed to what this nutritionist had to say. In my mind, I had chalked up all my diagnoses to corporate stress and travel.
>
> Guided by this logic, I proceeded to go on sabbatical for six months in 2016, thinking this would help me with a reset, and I would come back ready to take on the mantle of what I defined as success at the time. By spring 2018, my health was getting worse. I started to participate in a healthy eating program and watched some documentaries for homework. I ended up watching several: *Fat, Sick, and Nearly Dead*; *Forks Over Knives*; *What the Health*; *Cowspiracy*; and *Plant Pure Nation*. After watching them, I froze. I still remember how I felt. Everything that I had been told was wrong. I had a deep sense of disillusionment. I had lived for close to four decades, and I had

advanced education, and I didn't know about any of this. Clearly, I had not connected the dots!

Now I was being told that I could prevent and reverse disease, that I had some agency over what I had thought was my genetic destiny. I decided, "I'm going to jump right into it." On April 2, 2018, I started a whole-food, plant-based (WFPB), oil-free protocol, guided by Dr. Caldwell Esselstyn's book. Six months later, my health was great. My ovaries recovered, and my bloodwork and other tests were completely normal.

I helped my parents shift to a WFPB diet, and my mom reversed obesity, hypothyroidism, and hypertension, and no longer suffered from arthritis symptoms. She got off her medications within three months. My father, who had advanced kidney disease, didn't have to go back to the hospital for dialysis after a few months on the WFPB diet. His creatinine level, which was sky-high, came down to low single digits, not entirely normal, but still miraculous for someone who had needed dialysis. He was able to go back to eating fruits he loved but had shunned since he was diagnosed with diabetes, like mango. Imagine! He lived in India, surrounded by fruit orchards, and he had been told he couldn't eat fruit anymore. Now, he was ecstatic. Unfortunately, COVID-19 took him away from us in April 2020, but I'm looking at the silver lining. I'm glad that for the last few years of his life, he was healthier and happier.

Switching to a plant-based lifestyle reshaped my personality and life goals in a profound manner. My interpersonal and professional landscape is now evolving to be more aligned with my value system. Despite life's challenges—including that of complicated grief and loss during the global pandemic—I find myself more resilient than ever before.

Bob and Fran's story

Bob and Fran German are a couple in their eighties who are passionate teachers of healthy lifestyle and aging. I was inspired by the energy and vitality they showed, and by their story of healing. In 1992, Fran was diagnosed with myasthenia gravis, a neuromuscular autoimmune disease that causes severe muscle weakness. She said, "For fourteen years, I was very sick. I had many instances where I was unable to work, unable to speak, and unable to hold my head up. All doctors would do was give me medications. They gave me no hope to get better; I was told that my disease would shorten my lifespan and I would be on medication for the rest of my life."

In 2003, Fran and Bob started attending a local myasthenia gravis support group. This was the first time Fran had met other people with the same disorder. She notes, "I tried to be as healthy as I could, I exercised, practiced Tai Chi and Qi Gong. I thought I was eating healthy; for example, chicken white meat, and staying away from junk food. When I went to the support group, I saw that many of the people were very ill, with multiple diseases. And at the support group, what were they serving? They often had chips, soft drinks, and all kinds of junk food."

Fran indicated that at one of the support group meetings, "A nutritionist presented a program showing how even something as innocuous as white meat chicken compromised the immune system. He recommended that people with autoimmune diseases go on a whole-food, plant-based diet. He suggested that we read *The China Study* by T. Colin Campbell and *Diet for a New America* by John Robbins."

Bob and Fran had never thought about food as medicine, but they followed the nutritionist's recommendation and read the two books. Afterward, they immediately switched to a WFPB diet. Fran continued to follow up with her medical provider, and as her symptoms improved, her medications were adjusted. She initially had some difficulty getting off the prednisone that she had taken for several years. She subsequently consulted with a plant-based physician, who explained that prednisone shuts down the adrenals. Fran said, "He told me, 'First, I have to build up your adrenals and then take you down off the prednisone very slowly.' Since I got off the prednisone, I have not had any symptoms of myasthenia gravis, and have not been on any medication for sixteen years."

Bob shared that around the time they were learning about WFPB nutrition, he was diagnosed with renal cell carcinoma. He underwent cryoablation surgery and was warned by his doctor that his cancer could come back. Bob said that on the drive back home after his surgery, "We both made a commitment to go to a strict whole-food, plant-based diet and to do our best with it. We felt we needed a lifestyle change."

Since being plant-based, Bob and Fran remain active and exercise regularly. They enjoy plenty of food, while maintaining a healthy weight. Bob said, "We've always been foodies. We love to travel the world and eat different foods. Now we've become plant-based foodies."

Bob and Fran are passionate about the power of nutrition and lifestyle to support youthful aging. Bob said, "We took charge of our health. We now see doctors who are tuned into healthy eating and exercise and mindfulness." Through their YouTube channel, book, newsletter, and coaching, they support others to live active and healthy lives.

These stories, along with those of many others I interviewed, exemplify how we can take charge of our health through plant-based nutrition, an empowered mindset, and a healthful lifestyle. Although aging and death are inevitable parts of being human, through our lifestyle and nutrition choices, we have the potential to live and age more healthfully, youthfully, and vibrantly. We are not solely at the mercy of our family history, our genes, or an inevitable decline with aging; we have a say in our health and wellness. That realization is deeply empowering and is available to each of us.

Action Steps

You too can take charge of your health! Take the action steps that follow to increase your health empowerment:

- **Assess your health.** Explore these questions to take stock of your current level of health and wellness.
  - o How healthy do you consider yourself to be? (Not healthy, somewhat healthy, very healthy, extremely healthy?)
  - o Do you have any significant medical problems or symptoms that negatively impact your life?
  - o Have you had bloodwork or other preventive tests within the past year or so? (If not, are you due for a health check-up?) What did the results indicate?
  - o How would you rate your energy level? (Low, moderate, high?)
  - o Do you currently engage in healthy lifestyle practices?

- Eating predominantly or solely whole plant foods
- Reducing or eliminating highly processed foods, animal products, and added oils and sugar
- Active lifestyle and exercise
- Stress management and mindfulness
- Getting adequate sleep and rest
- Pleasurable and meaningful activities
- Time with loved ones
- Empowering self-talk

- **What changes do you want to make to improve your health and/or increase empowerment over your health?**
  o What lifestyle practices would you like to add or increase?
  o How might you benefit from cleaning up your diet and incorporating more nutrient-dense whole plant foods?
  o Are there new plant-based recipes or foods you want to try?
  o How might you change your self-talk to be more positive, self-compassionate, and empowering?
  o Are there books or other educational resources you want to check out?
  o Have you let your healthcare providers know your commitment to a healthy lifestyle, including plant-based nutrition, and asked if they will support you with this?

- **Set your action plan.** Now that you've assessed your health and lifestyle, choose a few changes you would like to start with, and set a date and plan for starting. Write your plan in your calendar or journal.
  o NOTE: Remember to consult with a qualified physician or healthcare professional if you plan to make significant changes in your diet or lifestyle, particularly if you have a medical condition. Shifting to a plant-based diet can improve certain health conditions (especially heart disease, high cholesterol, high blood pressure, and Type 2 diabetes) to the point that you may need to decrease or eliminate medications; it is important that this is monitored by a qualified professional. In addition, it is important that medications not be started, stopped, or changed without consultation and guidance from your medical provider.

o If you wish to consult with a healthcare professional who specializes in plant-based nutrition and/or lifestyle medicine, listings of providers are available on the websites of the American College of Lifestyle Medicine (ACLM), Plantrician.org, and PCRM.[36]

Taking charge of your health can free you to enjoy a more fulfilling, authentic, and meaningful life. It is empowering to see how each aspect of mind-body-spirit wellness connects with and impacts the other aspects in a multitude of ways. The next chapter discusses the inspiring awakening experience described by many vegans. Specifically, the realization that we are all truly connected: with each other, all sentient beings, and Mother Earth.

CHAPTER 8

DISCOVER YOUR INTERCONNECTEDNESS WITH LIFE

"Animals are my friends . . . and I don't eat my friends."

—George Bernard Shaw

"Martin Luther King taught us all nonviolence. I was told to extend nonviolence to the mother cow and her calf."

—Dick Gregory

"The greatness of a nation and its moral progress can be judged by the way its animals are treated."

—Mahatma Gandhi

My vegan awakening

When I became vegetarian (and later vegan), my willingness—and determination—to commit to this new lifestyle surprised me. My determination was fueled by an inner knowing that this was the "right thing" to do—ethically, nutritionally, and ecologically. As a former daily meat eater and comfort food seeker, I hadn't seen this transformation coming. It seemed spiritually guided, the way this life-affirming ethic and lifestyle unfolded in my life. Now I was truly living by foundational spiritual principles, like treating others as I would want to be treated and honoring my own body as a temple. This new way of living was uplifting and fulfilling—not a sacrifice, as I might have previously thought.

Spirituality has been a strong foundation in my life. I remember having a conversation with God at age four, standing in my backyard after Sunday School, looking at the sky, and full of questions I wanted to ask. I don't remember the questions, or receiving any answers, but I do remember having a sense of being connected to something mysterious, wise, and powerful, something far beyond the mundane. Throughout my life, I have had times of struggling with doubts and times of being distant from any faith, but I've always come back to following a spiritual path and trying to live by the guidance and principles that illuminated this path.

Once I was no longer consuming animal flesh and instead was nourished by plants from the bounty of nature, I felt in deeper alignment spiritually. Over time, I learned to trust my intuition more fully and to extend my compassion more widely. Living with greater *ahimsa*, the principle of nonviolence and non-harm to other sentient beings, felt more peaceful. Everything began to feel more integrated: my mind, body, spirit, as well as my connection to the divine and nature.

I have always loved the beauty of the outdoors, but now experience a greater sense of awe and mystery, along with times of guidance seemingly expressed through nature's creatures—whether it is a bluebird, butterfly, eagle, deer, or dragonfly that comes across my path in an unexpected or dramatic way. I now have a more poignant appreciation for the fact that we are all part of something larger, and that our well-being is interconnected with all life. In ways that are very tangible and obvious, as well as ways that seem more ethereal and mystical, my mind-body-spirit well-being is tethered to the flourishing of our planet and all its beings.

We are all interconnected

Spiritual experiences and a sense of interconnectedness came up quite often in my surveys and interviews with vegans. Not everyone identified spirituality right up front; slightly less than half endorsed "spiritual awakening or deepening" in a question that asked participants about the positive changes that came with being vegan. However, in open-ended responses to the survey and interviews, themes of spiritual and transcendent experiences came up again and again. For example, when asked about their emotional and spiritual experiences with a vegan lifestyle, several respondents made comments such as:

- "I now feel at one with the universe and all beings."
- "I feel connected to and appreciative of all living species."

- "I'm able to listen to my intuition and my heart more fully now."
- "I have a clear sense that we are all interconnected."
- "A fog has been lifted. I now experience a deeper connection to Spirit."

Those who participated in the survey came from a wide variety of religious and spiritual backgrounds, including some who were atheist and who did not resonate with the concept of spirituality at all. Despite differing backgrounds and beliefs, many described experiences of interconnectedness, intuitive guidance, appreciation, awe, spiritual awakening or deepening, moral alignment, and/or universal love as part of their vegan journey. The following is a sampling of survey responses that illustrate these themes.

Spiritual deepening

"I feel more spiritual now that I don't have to take a life to live a life."

"I had not really believed in God before . . . but now appreciate the miracle of life and the interwoven aspects of our bodies and the planet and understand there to be a higher power."

"What began as a logical thing to do after learning about animal cruelty over time turned into a spiritual journey, which was a surprising gift."

"Following a plant-based lifestyle deepens my connection with nature and the divine."

"My spirituality is deeply connected to my being vegan. All life on this planet is sacred."

Greater connectedness

"I feel that I am connected to my higher self and all living beings, we are all part of God's creation, we are one energy."

"I feel at ease with my choices and more in tune with the interconnectedness of everything."

"Finally, I am able to eat clean and in alignment with my personal ethics of 'do no harm.' I am clearer, more confident, much more deeply connected on an emotional and spiritual level. Consuming animal products dulled my senses. I now have greater empathy for all sentient beings and feel more connected to the interconnectedness of all things. This is what spirituality means to me . . . deep interconnectedness with the divine light and love in all living beings."

"Since becoming vegan, I experience the connection to others, animals, plants, and nature; increased sensitivity and intuitive awareness; and a much greater ease and expansion of love. A true awakening on every level."

"I feel a deeper connection with the world than I did before becoming vegan. I can see how all things are interconnected. The soil is a mirror of our health."

"I'm living in harmony with the web of life and doing the least harm possible to sustain my body and health."

Universal love and oneness

"I experience greater clarity of the concept of universal love and oneness. A vegan lifestyle is the only thing that will heal everything: human health, climate change, all the issues humans are dealing with today. Being vegan is the next stage of human evolution."

"The most significant impact I have experienced emotionally, spiritually, and socially is that WE ARE ALL ONE. I am at peace knowing that I no longer contribute to the suffering of other beings and the environment."

"It has allowed me to be more connected to nature as a whole and to understand my role on this planet. This has made me more compassionate toward animals but also toward people. I feel more peaceful, compassionate, empathetic, loving, and connected with the planet."

Compassion and ethics

"With awareness comes responsibility, and with responsibility comes a constant weight. There is nothing that I am more certain of than that being vegan is the 'right' way to live, an evolved and enlightened path through life, a more compassionate and charitable way to employ the life with which we have been blessed. In a world fraught with uncertainties, veganism is truth."

"My daily life is filled with peace, compassion, and equanimity, knowing that I am not harming other sentient beings. Knowing that veganism is the only path to living a true spiritual life of *ahimsa*."

"Being vegan allows me to live in alignment with my values and ahimsa, which has deepened my connection with the earth."

"Awakening to the truth that all life is spiritually connected and deserves respect has brought a sense of unity and peace. Once I consciously understood the full truth of animal exploitation and suffering, I could not 'unlearn' it. Although empathy for their plight continues to cause me emotional distress and despair, the benefit to my moral and spiritual sense of well-being outweighs any negatives."

"Veganism is a moral ethic that is a spiritual response to the imbalance on the planet. Veganism is an awakening . . . Mind-body-spirit healing and a vegan diet can create an environment and frequency in our bodies that will invite shifts that benefit All."

"Being vegan means living in alignment with my values and morals as someone who wants to leave all beings and the planet itself a better world when I'm gone. Knowing I am contributing to the net good: for animals, for the environment, for justice. I am zero percent spiritual, and I feel like a rejected outsider when vegans go on and on about spirituality as though it is a prerequisite to being an ethical vegan—which it's not. I don't feel a need to create a mysticism around being vegan. I can still experience awe, in fact even more so without spiritual baggage slapped on it."

Spirituality, awakening, and transcendence

How can we understand this sense of interconnectedness, oneness, compassion, and moral alignment described by many of my vegan participants? These qualities are espoused by spiritual teachers, philosophers, and social reformers as higher expressions of our humanity, something to seek, cultivate, and nurture, for our own greatest well-being and for a healthier and more loving world. The following are some guiding frameworks to better understand and make sense of these qualities and experiences.

Expressions of spirituality

There is no widely agreed upon definition of *spirituality*. While some equate spirituality with a belief in God or participation in organized religion, others view it more generally as our search for deeper, ultimate meaning. Spirituality can be expressed and experienced in a variety of ways: traditional religious practices, including religious services, rituals, or prayer; time in nature; reflection and contemplation; meditation;

journaling; and/or yoga. Many see spirituality as a connection to dimensions beyond our limited mind and body, including the divine, spirit, and/or our higher self. Some may not relate to the idea of God, but feel a connection to nature, Mother Earth, and/or the universe. Others may embrace a spirituality without religious connotation that encompasses self-transcendence, contemplative wisdom, and moral alignment.

William James, considered to be "the father of American psychology," examined the diversity of spiritual expressions in his seminal 1902 book, *The Varieties of Religious Experience*. He explored the inner, more personal aspects of how people experience spirituality. His work points to the centrality of spiritual and religious phenomena as part of our psychological make-up, spanning across time and cultures, and to the wide variety of forms these can take.[1]

Correlational research studies suggest that spiritual or religious involvement is associated with better physical and mental health, better health habits, improved stress management, resilience, increased social support, and lower risk of depression.[2] However, negative expressions of religiosity, such as avoiding life difficulties through religion or viewing religion as a means to an end, are associated with *greater* depression.[3]

The neurobiology of awakening

Dr. Lisa Miller, author of *The Awakened Brain*, gives this description of spirituality:

> Many of us have had experiences we might describe as spiritual. A moment of deep connection with another being or in nature. A feeling of awe or transcendence. An experience of startling synchronicity or a time when a stranger showed up and did something that changed your life. A time you felt held or inspired or buoyed up by something greater than yourself—a higher power perhaps, but also nature or the universe or even the surge of connection at a concert or sporting event.[4]

Dr. Miller is a clinical psychology professor at Columbia University and director of the Spiritual Mind Body Institute. She and her colleagues have done fascinating research on spirituality, depression, and the neural circuitry of the brain. Dr. Miller argues that we each have the neurological capability to be in touch with a greater reality beyond ourselves:

Whether or not we participate in a spiritual practice or adhere to a faith tradition, whether or not we identify as religious or spiritual, our brain has a natural inclination toward and docking station for spiritual awareness. The awakened brain is the neural circuitry that allows us to see the world more fully and thus enhance our individual, societal, and global well-being.[5]

Dr. Miller's interest and research in spirituality came out of her work as a clinical psychologist, where she found that spiritual experiences often played an important role in emotional resilience and healing but tended to be overlooked or minimized by the mental health profession. Her collaborative research, which included MRI (magnetic resonance imaging) scans of the brain, found that spirituality is reflected in our brain neurocircuitry. Those reporting higher spirituality showed healthier and more robust neural structures. This greater neural health was particularly evident in parts of the brain that have been found to be vulnerable to "withering" or deteriorating in people with depression. Her research found that spirituality protected against future depression, particularly in those with high genetic risk.[6]

Drawing on fMRI (functional magnetic resonance imaging) technology to map brain responses, Dr. Miller and her colleagues sought to discover how we could activate the benefits of spirituality. They found that we have two modes of awareness: achieving awareness and awakened awareness. *Achieving awareness* focuses on organizing and managing our lives so that we can meet our desires and needs. It helps us direct energy and focus toward reaching goals. This mode of awareness helps us get things done. However, we can get out of balance, focusing narrowly on "achieving" and losing sight of the bigger picture. When achieving awareness is overused, it can change the structure of the brain and contribute to depression, anxiety, and stress, as well as a tendency toward addictive behaviors.[7]

Awakened awareness involves different neural pathways than achieving awareness. It is activated by transcendent experiences, connection, compassion, curiosity, awe, or wonder. This mode of awareness gives us a larger perspective, attunement to the relationships between events in our lives, and greater receptivity to creative insights. Rather than being stuck in familiar ruts of perception, we can see a bigger picture. Dr. Miller argues that to truly flourish, we need *both* achieving and awakened awareness to inform and guide our actions.[8]

As we cultivate our capacity for awakened awareness, we become more aware of our impact on others and the world and can make choices that contribute not only to our own well-being but also to the greater good. Neurobiology research teaches us that we can resculpt our neural pathways through how we focus our attention.[9] By attuning to our connections with others and the world, noticing synchronicities, and nurturing mindful, heartful, and spiritual qualities, we can deepen our awakened awareness. The experiences shared by many of my vegan research participants seem reflective of an awakened awareness that recognizes the larger connections between self and all beings and that is guided by altruism and compassion.

Self-Transcendence

The spiritual and unitive experiences described by my vegan participants can also be understood through the lens of *transcendence*. You may have heard of psychologist Abraham Maslow, who is well known for his Hierarchy of Needs model. This model of growth starts with meeting our foundational physiological and safety needs, followed by our needs for love and self-esteem, and culminates in self-actualization (the full realization of our intellectual, social, and creative potential). Less well-known are Maslow's later teachings, which included transcendence as the ultimate evolution in human development and flourishing, a step beyond self-actualization.

The book *Transcend*, by Scott Barry Kaufman, Ph.D., offers an in-depth exploration of Maslow's teachings, including unpublished works from later in his life. Dr. Kaufman describes transcendence as "harnessing all that you are in the service of realizing the best version of yourself so you can help raise the bar for the whole of humanity."[10] Transcendent experiences fall on a continuum, ranging from more common experiences, such as being absorbed in a book or artwork, to life-changing experiences, such as sensing one's interconnectedness with a larger whole. In between these extremes are experiences such as mindful presence, gratitude, awe, wonder, and love.[11] Kaufman states that at its most intense level, transcendence can encompass "a feeling of complete unity with everything . . . including other humans (the social environment), as well as all of existence, nature, and the cosmos (the spatial environment)."[12]

Transcendent consciousness is associated with more positive mental health, improved relationships, reduced fear of death, and better physical health, as well as increased altruistic behaviors.[13] However, Kaufman explains that "transcenders" (those dedicated to "becoming better human beings for others, as well as for themselves" per Maslow)[14] may not always feel happy or be motivated by happiness. They may experience heights of joy or rapture, but also may experience a "cosmic sadness" as they hold a vision for the world that is not yet realized.[15] Kaufman stresses the importance, based on Maslow's teachings, of meeting our more basic needs and building a strong, integrated sense of self as a foundation for *healthy* self-transcendence. Emotions that may accompany self-transcendence include gratitude, awe, compassion, appreciation, inspiration, and admiration.[16]

Veganism and spirituality

Themes such as spirituality, awakening, and transcendence are difficult to define, yet are integral and integrating aspects of the mystery and fabric of life. These qualities of our human experience can bring out what is best in us and give greater meaning and fulfillment to our existence. Experiences of awakening, unity, and interconnectedness may be cultivated through spirituality or religion, as well as through practices such as mindfulness, meditation, gratitude, and compassion.

How are these experiences associated with the vegan journey? Not all vegans report these types of experiences; however, they came up often enough in my research, and in other sources on veganism and spirituality, to know that this isn't just an isolated phenomenon.[17] Some of my participants described their experiences of interconnectedness as part of a larger spiritual journey that led them to veganism. These vegans had already been doing inner growth work, including meditation or spiritual exploration, to become better versions of themselves. Along that path, they discovered veganism, which closely aligned with their core spiritual beliefs. Some, who didn't identify with spirituality or religion, strongly resonated with moral values of compassion and kindness, and becoming vegan emerged as an expression of these values.

For many, their decision to become vegan seemed to open the door to greater spiritual awareness and depth. They described experiencing psychological and physiological changes once they were no longer consuming animals that led to a greater awareness of how they were connected to all sentient beings and all of life. When we honor our moral and ethical values by not eating animals, we have less we need to defend against. This may allow us to be more open to seeing our connections with one another, all animals, our planet, and the universe.

Thus, veganism can be connected to spirituality and transcendence in a number of ways. Some of these interconnections are highlighted next.

Veganism is a tangible expression of spiritual, ethical, and moral values.

At its very core, veganism is a philosophy and practice that seeks to avoid exploitation, harm, and cruelty to all sentient beings. It's not a diet per se, but rather a lifestyle based on the compassionate and ethical treatment of animals. The commitment to live with greater kindness and less harm to others is at the heart of most ethical guidelines, spiritual traditions, and social reform movements. Victoria Moran, best-selling author and founder of Main Street Vegan Academy, shares how spirituality and veganism are fundamentally connected in her life: "Being Vegan gives me an opportunity to translate what's come to me via spiritual teachings into something real and palpable right here on earth."[18]

Although many spiritual and religious traditions underscore the importance of compassion, non-harm, and nonviolence, in practice this rarely includes *all* sentient beings. The concepts of compassion and non-harm are mostly applied only to other humans (and then often only those who are "like us"). Rarely do those of us in spiritual circles consider how our food choices contribute to harm and violence. However, some wise teachers argue that the optimal state for humanity is to live as pure vegetarians—pointing, for example, to the original Garden of Eden, where a solely plant-based diet was consumed. These values are also illustrated in the Bible's book of Daniel, which shares how Daniel and his friends refused the rich, animal-based meals offered by the king and flourished with plant foods such as vegetables and legumes.[19]

Many religious and spiritual traditions, such as Buddhism, Yogic traditions, Hinduism, Jainism, as well as some sects of Christianity, Judaism, and Islam, have historically promoted a vegetarian lifestyle as an expression of compassion and/or purity.[20] While we don't see the practice of vegetarianism or veganism widely applied in most religions currently, one can argue that a vegan lifestyle is a true embodiment of spiritual teachings. This is particularly true at the present time, when intensive animal agriculture causes more suffering and greater environmental destruction than at any other time in history.

In the book *The Inner Art of Vegetarianism*, author Carol J. Adams teaches that a vegetarian or vegan lifestyle can be considered a spiritual practice. She describes *spiritual vegetarianism* as "the practice of living from a diet comprised wholly of vegetables, grains, fruits, nuts, and seeds," which is founded on a desire for wholeness, a commitment to nonviolence, and the acknowledgement of our interconnectedness with nature and all beings. Adams explains that vegan ethics and lifestyle synergistically support and align with other spiritual practices, such as meditation, yoga, prayer, and reflection.[21]

The metaphysics of food

The study of metaphysics teaches us that all matter has a frequency or vibration, including the foods we consume. When you consider modern animal agriculture practices, in which most animals live and die under incredible levels of stress and fear, it seems likely that the stress chemicals in their bodies would have a negative impact on our mind, body, and spirit when we ingest them.[22] In addition, because toxins become concentrated in animal flesh, the unnatural diets fed to factory farmed animals—laden with antibiotics, hormones, pathogens, and pesticides—can cause toxins to also build up in our bodies and brains. Dr. Will Tuttle, author of *The World Peace Diet*, explains, "We are rediscovering what Pythagoras taught us: that eating animal foods has negative effects on our consciousness." Pythagoras, the ancient Greek philosopher who is famous for his Pythagorean theorem, advocated a vegetarian lifestyle as foundational to mind-body-spirit wellness, as well as to a more peaceful co-existence.[23]

The links between harm to animals and humans

The wisdom conveyed through books such as *The World Peace Diet* by Dr. Tuttle, *The Phoenix Zones* by Dr. Hope Ferdowsian, and *How to End Injustice Everywhere* by Dr. Melanie Joy teach us that justice, peace, and well-being for humans is inextricably intertwined with our treatment of animals.[24] Dr. Ferdowsian captures this interrelationship when she states that we must address "the deepest origins of discrimination and abuse—including violence directed at animals. If we neglect any branch of violence, it can take root like a metastatic form of cancer, spreading across the invisible lines we've created and placing us all at risk."[25]

Many great thinkers from earlier times, ranging from Pythagoras to Leonardo DaVinci to Leo Tolstoy, have argued that true peace, justice, and enlightenment will occur only when we end violence toward both human *and* non-human animals. In addition to the opening quotes of this chapter from Gandhi, Dick Gregory, and George Bernard Shaw, consider these wise reflections from historical figures:

> For as long as men massacre animals, they will continue to kill each other. Indeed, he who sows the seed of murder and pain cannot reap joy and love.—Pythagoras

> He who is cruel to animals becomes hard also in his dealings with man. We can judge the heart of a man by his treatment of animals.—Immanuel Kant

> I have from an early age abjured the use of meat, and the time will come when men such as I will look upon the murder of animals as they now look upon the murder of men.—Leonardo DaVinci

> By killing animals for food, a person suppresses in himself the higher spiritual sentiments—compassion and mercy for other living creatures, similar to him—and, stifling himself, he hardens his heart.—Leo Tolstoy

> When you feel the suffering of every living thing in your own heart, that is consciousness.—From the Bhagavad Gita

Our connection to the planet

Spiritual teachings encourage us to be good stewards of the earth upon which we live. Our food choices, purchases, daily habits, societal practices, and industries all have an impact on the health of our environment. Intensive animal agriculture is the greatest contributor to destruction of the environment, including deforestation, species extinction, pollution, greenhouse gas emissions, and the depletion of resources. The devastation of our environment disproportionately affects Indigenous peoples, minorities, and those with less economic power. Our own well-being and survival are strongly intertwined with our treatment of Mother Earth, as is evidenced by increasing extreme weather events, droughts, wildfires, floods, rising sea levels, pollution, water shortages, and soil depletion. These events are contributing to the loss of livelihoods—and lives. The reverse is also true: As we care for and nurture our planet and all sentient beings on it, we too are nurtured and more likely to flourish.

As beautifully expressed by one of my research participants, vegan empowerment coach, Mariquita Solis:

> "Veganism connects with every part of existence. In nature, we can feel our connection with every living being, every tree, every grain of sand. When I put my hand in the soil, I realize that this is a living force. The soil, the trees, and our lives are all connected. Our Earth has been disregarded, and this mirrors our sense of disconnection."

Mariquita serves in leadership roles for her church's Animal Ministry and Healthy Living Group and is on the board of Earth Care Ministry. She explains,

> "These ministries are all tied together, and I try to help people see this. Our choice whether or not to eat animals affects all these areas. This is the question for us to think about: 'Are you eating peace or are you eating pain and suffering?'"

Becoming aware of our interconnectedness with all Life, and the call to compassionate living that comes with this, are foundational and life-changing insights for many vegans. Next, I share the stories of Michelle, Heather, and Pat, who each illustrate how these themes touched their lives.

Michelle's story

Michelle Schaefer became vegetarian in her twenties and went vegan a couple of years later after reading *Diet for a New America* by John Robbins. She didn't eat healthfully during college and graduate school and was hospitalized after going on a very low-fat diet for several months. After over seven years of veganism, she lapsed back to eating dairy products. Following her father's death in 2016, she became motivated to return to a vegan lifestyle.

> Initially I craved cheese, but I made a deal with myself. I said, 'Okay, Michelle, you can eat all the dairy you want, but you have to watch a sixty-second dairy video before you eat it, so you can't deny what you are doing.' That stopped it immediately. PETA's *Dairy in 60 Seconds* rewired my brain.

Michelle added, "The horrific video association meant I didn't crave cheese anymore. It might not work that way for everyone, but it was neuronal anarchy for me." Michelle went on to write a Meatless Monday article for her local paper and start a vegan meet-up group. Now she writes freelance, as well as for *bUneke* magazine, and works as a Reader Ambassador for *VegNews Magazine*. Michelle shared how veganism has impacted her ethically and emotionally:

> I came alive at age 47. I'd never felt so vibrant. When my behavior truly aligned with the values that always had been there, I felt a wonderful sense of peace, jubilation, and liberation. After a while, my awareness expanded. First it was the plastic my arugula came in and fast fashion—then larger issues like institutionalized racism, ageism, ableism, and so much more became part of my consciousness. One core value—wanting to end animal suffering—led to an entirely new way of thinking. Awareness of oppression is, for better or worse, ever-expanding. While awareness is good, I've discovered that balance is required. As it says in Ecclesiastes, "In much wisdom is much grief. Those that increaseth knowledge increaseth sorrow."[26]
>
> Many new vegans become depressed when they learn about all the harm done to animals. I completely get that, but that was not something that happened to me in the beginning. I was so relieved to know that I was doing the very best I could to no longer contribute to that kind of suffering. I just felt joy—so much joy—so much peace

and happiness. Just a vibrancy that I had never experienced before. I became more *me*. It felt like, "Wow, this is who I've been from the womb!" At age 47, everything was finally able to come together. It brought such relief and jubilance. I was and remain so deeply grateful that I get to be a vegan on this journey.

Michelle has learned along the way to take better care of herself with healthier nutrition, as well as general self-care. She said, "Overall, I have more stamina and feel better now at fifty-three than I felt at twenty-one." She added,

> I don't want *any* bodies to suffer, those precious, innocent, sweet animals who have never done anything to anybody . . . their bodies, hearts, and minds suffer all the time. I hate that. I honor their bodies, *and* I am learning to honor my own body. I don't need to be a martyr. It does not have to be either-or.

Michelle said that she identifies with Buddhist philosophies, but elaborated:

> Actually, veganism is my religion. It's a set of beliefs that guides everything I do. Don't get me wrong, I have a feeling there is some sort of higher power. I refer to her as Mother Goddess. But with veganism, I don't have to imagine any ethereal being. If I want to see Hell, all I have to do is watch a factory farm video. There's no question for anyone—unless they are a genuine psychopath—that what goes on in factory farming is morally repulsive and that it would not be pleasing to *any* god. There's no mystery involved. Conversely, if you watch videos of a rescued cow joyfully playing with a yoga ball, you get to see Heaven right here on earth.
>
> With factory farm or rescue sanctuary videos, we can see images of Hell or Heaven. We don't have to use our imagination. We don't need to go back to ancient times. Personally, I don't have to believe in anything other than kindness for veganism to feel like my religion. For me, veganism means personal joy and absolute freedom from the anxiety that came from years of loving animals *and* eating them. I mean, how can we say, "I love animals," while eating them? We would never say, "I love my neighbor," while simultaneously burning their house down. Veganism destroys that type of cognitive dissonance. The clarity it brings replaces the internal battle of cognitive dissonance with a garden of peace and purpose.

Heather's story

Heather is a health coach, grief coach, and yoga enthusiast. She said, "I've always been a deeply empathetic person. I cried when I went fishing with my grandparents, and they caught the fish. I felt the animals' feelings so deeply as a child. I still ate meat, because I had to do what my parents said until I was old enough to rebel." She became vegetarian at around age twelve or thirteen. She had some lapses from vegetarianism in her twenties, when she first got married, due to family pressures, but later resumed a meat-free lifestyle.

> When I went back to eating animal products out of trying to appease others, I felt bad emotionally, I felt sad and distressed. When these animals suffer for their whole life, and they die these horrible deaths, that energy goes into their body. Then when we consume them, we are also consuming that energy of fear, anger, and sadness. I believe that the action of eating meat numbs the soul to things it should feel.

Five years ago, after seeing a social media post about the dairy and egg industries, she became vegan. She said:

> Sometimes I'm ashamed that I haven't been vegan for my whole life. I'm 45. I should have known better way sooner. But I have to give myself grace, because I truly didn't know. And if I did, I would have made a better choice. I think most people know inside their heart. If you look at most children, they have love and compassion for animals. They want to protect and love any little animal. But it's the conditioning of society, the role modeling of adults that changes the way we feel about animals. The animals become a product. But that's not how we're born.
>
> Being vegan calms my soul. It makes me feel at home, in alignment with the whole universe. Even when other people say negative things to me, it still doesn't change that calm water inside of me. Because I know that I'm doing what I can do. I'm not contributing with my money and with what I put in my body to animal suffering. I've never felt so spiritually aligned as the last five years or so of my life. Because I'm not contributing to harm and suffering to another being. Love, compassion, and empathy for other beings is at the core of most religions. There's a common thread. But people don't notice that common thread—because it would challenge their lifestyle.

I feel that it's been a great aid in my spiritual development to be vegan. I don't see myself as "holier than thou." No, it feels more like I'm finally living the way I should. It's hard to explain to people about the spiritual impact that being vegan can have on you. As someone who has always been sensitive and empathic, I can't imagine ever going back. I can't imagine sacrificing my emotional wellness or the spiritual alignment that I feel in living this way. I hope to inspire others toward veganism, to be a light that draws people and meets them where they are, with compassion.

Pat's story

Pat LaStrapes' path to veganism started after his sister's death in 2003, when he adopted her white German Shepherd. Prior to this, he describes himself as a "full-fledged carnivore." He had always loved animals, however, and a special bond was formed with this dog. He said, "I began to see how intelligent and incredible she was. We had a great relationship, and I learned a lot from her." Over time, he began to think more about the sentience of all beings, and gradually shifted his diet, first to pescatarian, then vegetarian, and finally vegan, over about a ten-year period. He said, "Once you pull back the curtain and see, you can't go back. Now I try to be kind to all beings. I take spiders outside, rather than kill them."

Pat noted that spirituality is an important part of his life, adding, "Veganism and the spiritual path go hand in hand." He studies the teachings of many religions, including Buddhism, Daoism, Jainism, and Christianity. He tries to live in the moment, "being open to the lessons of the day." He reports increased inner reflection since becoming vegan: "I'm more conscious of the ripple effects of my actions. Looking back, I see that I was callous and egotistical at times. Where I am now is many galaxies apart from where I was."

Pat acknowledged that sometimes he feels deep regret about past choices, which brings guilt and grief. He feels he is now more authentic and honest, quicker to own when he has done something wrong and to apologize. As a result, he experiences "more fruitful and happy relationships."

I have less inner conflict now, and I feel good about that. Now I live consistently with my values. The natural law is written on our hearts, a silent thing that speaks to us. If something feels as right as rain, then, perhaps, it is right as rain. I know, at the deepest level of consciousness, that I am doing the right thing. This brings me a measure of peace.

As reflected in these stories, veganism is an embodied expression of our deepest moral values and spiritual teachings. As we eat more cleanly and live more compassionately, veganism can awaken in us the realization of our interconnectedness with all living beings and the larger universe in which we live. This awareness can bring great joy and peace, as it lifts us out of the disconnection, isolation, and alienation so prominent in our current times, to a sense that we are indeed part of something beautiful, magical, and wonderful. In opening to awe and wonder, compassion, and universal love, we also awaken to our greater humanity. We realize that our well-being is intertwined with the well-being of all, that in the end, they are one and the same.

Action Steps

How can we cultivate our sense of interconnectedness with our higher knowing, all beings, and the natural world? The following are some exercises to tap into self-transcendence. Practice those that resonate with you.

- **Meditate regularly.** In order to access our wiser, more awakened brain, we need to be able to quiet our minds. Often, our minds are racing with an ongoing running commentary of thoughts, ruminations, and judgments. Meditation practices teach us how to witness the activities of our mind, and in doing so, become more mindfully present and less reactive. Generally, meditation involves bringing our awareness to a focal point, such as the breath, a mantra, an image, or physical sensations, and continually returning our attention back to this focal point. Having a regular meditation practice helps to rewire the brain so that we can experience less rumination, obsessiveness, and anxiety.[27] *Here is a simple mindful meditation practice, focused on the breath:*

o Set a timer for however long you want to meditate (five to ten minutes is fine if you are just getting started).

o Focus on the flow of your breath in and out until the timer goes off.

o Continually bring your focus back to your breath. If you are like most human beings, your mind is destined to wander. The practice is not so much about having a perfectly quiet mind (even many long-term meditators do not experience that), but rather about noticing when your mind has wandered and bringing your mind back to the breath. With practice, it becomes easier to recognize when your mind has wandered and bring it back.

o Keep a journal of your meditation practice, and note any changes in your moods, thinking, reactivity, awareness, and/or mindful presence in daily life.

- **Raise your vibration through what you eat.** As noted earlier, the foods we eat play a role in our consciousness. Eating dense animal foods (the products of fear, stress, violence, and death) affects us in ways that we may not fully realize until we take them off our plates. Nurture your mind, body, and spirit by eating more compassionately, sustainably, and healthfully, centering your nutrition on whole plant foods, including plenty of raw fruits and veggies. Consider going to your local farmers market, community garden, or community supported agriculture (CSA) for fresh, seasonal produce. Cultivate appreciation for the food you eat, reflecting on all that brings the food to your table: the sun, the soil, the rain; those who cultivate, grow, and harvest the crops; and those who transport and sell them. Keep a journal of your emotional, physical, and spiritual well-being as you make changes in your eating habits and mindset.

- **Recall a spiritual or transcendent experience in nature.** Think of a time that you were deeply moved or uplifted by the natural world. You may have felt touched by a higher power, awed or inspired by the beauty around you, or experienced guidance, a surprising synchronicity, or a message through some aspect of your experience. Maybe you had a transformative encounter with an animal. Reconnecting with these types of experiences can open the door to access greater peace, wisdom, and intuitive awareness, and give hope and perspective during difficult times. Step back into that experience and use all your senses to connect to it.

o   What do you see, feel, hear, sense?

o   As you connect with the memory and feelings of this experience, how does your awareness expand? What opens up for you?

o   How does this experience shift your perspective?

o   How can you bring this deeper awareness and presence into your daily life?

- **Animal Guide Meditation.** Follow the instructions below. If you like, you can listen to a recording of this meditation on my website.[28]

o   Find a comfortable place, where you will not be disturbed. After getting comfortable, close your eyes or soften your gaze. Focus on taking five slow, deep breaths, and start to quiet your mind and body.

o   Imagine yourself in a beautiful place in nature, ideally a place that brings a sense of peace, calm, and perhaps awe. It can be somewhere you have been before, or a place you create in your own imagination. Picture it, drawing on all your senses: the sights, sounds, textures, feelings, and smells.

o   Once you are comfortable in your peaceful place, invite your Animal Guide(s) to join you here. Invite any animals, of any species, that are here to help or guide you. Picture them as they join you in this beautiful place. Feel the support and the wisdom that they bring you.

o   Notice the special qualities and characteristics of your Animal Guide(s). What can you learn from these animals and their natural strengths? How can these unique qualities help, support, inspire, nurture, protect, or guide you? How might you integrate these qualities into your life?

o   If you are struggling with a question or challenge, ask your Animal Guide questions such as, "What do I need to know now?" "What is my next step?" or "What is best for me and for the greatest good?" Listen to any answers, noticing that they may come in the form of words, symbols, images, behaviors, or feelings.

o   When the conversation feels complete (for now), thank your Animal Guide, and if you wish, discuss plans to meet again. Say goodbye, let your peaceful place fade away, and come back to the present, back to the room where you are seated.

o   Write down anything you learned from this conversation, as well as how you felt during the encounter. Notice any sense of strengthened connection or awareness. Are there any actions you want to take, based on this experience?

Over the last several chapters, we've reviewed the *seven core transformations* uncovered through my vegan research. As you consider the transformative possibilities that you may experience with vegan living, what awarenesses are opening up for you? What changes do you feel called to make or deepen? Perhaps you wish to go further with some of the exercises and action steps that have been suggested so far. If you are like many of us, you may have experienced difficulties with starting or maintaining lifestyle changes in the past, and wonder, can you follow through? The next few chapters dive into how to move from awareness and awakening into meaningful action. Let's go on to Chapter Nine, where I share principles and tools for successful (and lasting) lifestyle change.

PART THREE

FROM AWAKENING
TO ACTION

CHAPTER 9

KEYS TO SUCCESSFUL LIFESTYLE CHANGE

"In order to change your behavior, the first thing you need to change is your mind."

—**James O. Prochaska**, Ph.D. and **Janice M. Prochaska**, Ph.D. in *Changing to Thrive* [1]

"Your behaviors are usually a reflection of your identity. What you do is an indication of the type of person you believe that you are—either consciously or nonconsciously."

—**James Clear** in *Atomic Habits* [2]

"Embrace mistakes as discoveries and use them to move forward."

—**BJ Fogg**, Ph.D. in *Tiny Habits* [3]

Preparing for change

We've covered seven amazing transformations that can unfold when you make the decision to leave animals off your plate and instead nourish your mind, body, and spirit with wholesome plant foods. With this lifestyle, you have the potential to create holistic well-being through honoring your values, widening your compassion, finding greater meaning and purpose, cultivating authentic fulfillment, nurturing meaningful connections, taking charge of your health, and realizing your interconnectedness with life. As you consider all the reasons for eating more plants and moving away from animal products, perhaps you're all in and ready to go. Or maybe you have some concerns about how this will work for you. How can you transition to a plant-powered lifestyle successfully? How will you handle any challenges you may face?

This chapter is for you, whether you are curious about experimenting with more plant-based meals, going all the way to a vegan lifestyle, or are already vegan but want to improve your life in some way. Maybe you want to increase your emotional or physical wellness, overcome a health issue, or feel more fulfilled and/or purposeful. Maybe you sense something is missing in your life and want to fill in the gaps to create holistic, compassionate, mind-body-spirit flourishing.

Whatever your goals may be, you will be embarking on a journey of change. We sometimes welcome change, while at other times we steadfastly resist it. The truth is that change is part of life. Sometimes it's forced on us by our circumstances, such as a health crisis, a tragedy, or a loss. And other times we proactively decide that it's time to make a change—to create a better life, to be more aligned with our core values, needs, and/or desires. Sometimes we have a sudden awakening, from something we read or hear about (e.g., a book such as this one) that leads us to decide it's time to change. Other times, the change is more gradual, from seeds that have been taking root over time.

Whatever has brought you to this place, now is a good time to ask yourself: "What changes do I want to make? What steps do I want to take to move forward?" Take some time to let these questions percolate as you review this chapter; it will guide you in clarifying your vision and goals while providing information about the process of making healthy and lasting change, so that you can be as successful as possible in moving toward your goals. You'll have the opportunity to do some in-depth exploration through questions, reflections, and action steps that prepare you for successful change.

In the limited space of this chapter, I'm aware that it may be difficult to do full justice to this topic, because the process of change could be a whole book in and of itself. And indeed, there are many books that offer a deep dive into how to change habits and create a healthier lifestyle.[4] I also won't be able to cover all the specifics of how to transition to a vegan lifestyle, although hopefully you will gain some insights for getting started. To learn more about the HOW of becoming plant-based or vegan, I highly recommend checking out some of the books listed in the Resources section in this book.

This chapter provides a starting guide or overview of general strategies to support you in *initiating* and *maintaining* successful lifestyle change. I will be focusing my message toward helping you transition to a plant-based or vegan lifestyle, but the ideas can be applied for any kind of lifestyle or behavior change. In the next chapter (Chapter Ten), I will discuss how to handle emotional and social challenges that you may face as a vegan, so that you can *thrive* with a plant-powered lifestyle.

The tips that I share in this chapter draw from my twenty-five years of experience as a psychologist helping clients create lifestyle change for greater emotional and physical wellness. I also draw on my own experience of transformation in many areas of my own life, including health habits, fitness, self-esteem, relationships, spirituality, and adopting a vegan lifestyle. In addition, I draw on insights offered by other experts in the field of lifestyle change, as well as the wisdom and experience of the vegans that I interviewed for this research.

For most of us, changing our lifestyle is a journey with many steps. It is often a process that occurs over time versus an overnight transformation (although they can certainly happen). The following are reflections and action steps for your vegan transformation journey. We will start by setting your intention and vision for change, then explore potential obstacles, and finally identify strategies and resources to successfully move toward your vision.

Create a plan

First, you need to determine what you want to change and what this will look like. It's also important to identify your motivations for change, your WHY. Next, you need a grounded action plan to achieve your goals. Reflect on the following questions to help set your plan for change, and record your responses in your journal.

1. **Assess where you are currently:** How are you feeling now, physically, mentally, emotionally, and spiritually?

2. **What parts of your life do you most want to improve?** What improvements in your health, emotional well-being, fulfillment, values alignment, spirituality, relationships, purpose, contribution, or other life areas would you like to experience? If you want to move toward a vegan or plant-based lifestyle, how might this help bring improvement in the areas you've identified?

3. **What behaviors do you want to change** to achieve greater well-being in these areas? What habits will you put into practice, and which old habits do you wish to stop?

4. **Assess your current mindset.** How can you empower, encourage, and support yourself to create these changes? Which negative self-messages tend to derail you? How can you cultivate more empowering self-messages?

5. **What would your life look like and feel like if you made these changes?** Create a vision and feel for a sense of what would be different if you reached your goals. What positives would ripple into other areas of your life?

6. **Connect a little deeper with your WHY for change.** What are your most compelling reasons for wanting to make a change? What is the driving force or vision that motivates you to move forward? Was there an epiphany you had, whether from this book or elsewhere? Is there an area of your life where you feel out of alignment? How will this change help you be more in alignment with the person you want to be? Write a statement that captures your most important reasons for change: *My WHY for making this change is* _____.

7. **What type of person do you envision yourself being?** What is the identity you want to cultivate as a result of these changes? Create a statement that reflects this identity. For example: *I am healthy, fit, and active; I live by my ethical values; I am purposeful and fulfilled; I am a person who lives and speaks my truth; I am a force for positive change in the world; I am a compassionate, healthy vegan.*

8. **Create clear goals and set your action plan.** Envisioning our dreams and goals can motivate us to get started, but for successful and lasting change, we also need a grounded plan with daily actions and habits. Drawing on your vision, create a clear plan to implement changes. You will fill in more details of this plan as you work on the additional exercises and reflections later in this chapter. However, you can create a starting plan, using the SMART goal-setting framework. SMART stands for Specific, Measurable, Achievable, Relevant, and Timebound, as discussed next.[5]

a. **Specific:** *What* specifically do you want to change? Also consider the *how*, *where*, *when*, and *who* for carrying this out. For example, if you want to eat more plant-based meals (your *what*), be specific about *how many* plant-based meals per day or week, and *when*, *where*, and *how* you will do this, as well as *who* will be involved to support you. If you want to go fully vegan, go through these same questions to gain clarity and pin down the specifics of how you will get started.

b. **Measurable:** How will you know that you've reached your goal? What specific changes will let you know?

c. **Achievable:** Is your goal realistic and attainable? It's fine if it seems like a bit of a stretch but consider whether it is truly doable. You may decide your goal is more achievable if you break it into smaller steps. *For example*: If you want to adopt a vegan lifestyle, but it feels too overwhelming to do at once, you may want to try a more gradual approach. You could start by incorporating several plant-based meals, then remove one animal product at a time, with the goal of removing all animal products over a specified timeframe.

d. **Relevant:** Is this change something that truly matters to you? Connect again with your WHY. Does the vision of reaching your goal inspire and motivate you?

e. **Timebound:** Set a specific timeframe for reaching your goal. There is something about setting a target date that helps us to follow through. For example, if you plan to adopt a vegan lifestyle, what is your date for that to go into effect? Set a target date for reaching your goal and write it down in your journal or calendar.

Identify your obstacles

Whenever we make lifestyle changes, we are likely to encounter some difficulties. For one, there is a learning curve with any change. There is new information to learn, new habits to cultivate, and old habits to eliminate. In addition, we have to deal with our social context. Will the people in our life be supportive of our changes, or will they (wittingly or unwittingly) undermine us? And let's be honest; when it comes to making changes, even the changes we really want to make, we sometimes undermine ourselves through old habits, fears, or limiting beliefs. Inventory the possible challenges that could block you from the goals you have set. You may not be prepared for every challenge; some may surprise you. I encourage you to be kind to yourself through the process of working toward your goals, and to view any setbacks as an opportunity to learn and grow.

The following are some questions to help you consider where you may face challenges, so you can set a plan to address these. It is helpful to write your responses in your journal. In the sections that follow, for the sake of clarity, I will specifically focus on the challenges you may face in adopting a *vegan lifestyle*. If your goal is something different (for example, to incorporate more plant-based meals, eliminate added sugar or ultra-processed foods from your diet, or start a meditation practice), you can apply these same questions to uncover potential barriers or challenges.

Practical challenges

What is most difficult for you in making this change? What roadblocks do you anticipate in the day-to-day reality of moving toward your goal? For example: *I'm not a good cook; I don't know any vegan or plant-based recipes; I don't know which plant-based or vegan options can replace my favorite foods; I'm addicted to cheese and can't imagine giving it up; How will I find vegan foods when I travel?; I don't know how to get my key nutrients; I'm not sure where to purchase vegan, cruelty-free products.* In my vegan transition, my top three challenges were: finding appealing breakfast options that were egg-free; making delicious vegan baked goods; and replacing cosmetics with cruelty-free options. Make a list of three to five practical challenges that you anticipate.

Social and family challenges

Your social network can be your biggest support in healthy change—or your biggest obstacle. For those transitioning to a vegan lifestyle, learning how to navigate social situations and gatherings may be one of the most daunting hurdles. Consider your current relationships and social network to identify possible challenges you may face.

Think about your family and close friends. How supportive are they likely to be of your goal? What concerns might they have? How can you educate them and bring them on board as an ally, so that they understand why this change is important to you? How would you like them to support you? What social gatherings, traditions, and holidays do you attend that center around animal foods? How might you handle these situations? What new traditions and foods can you introduce that support your new lifestyle? How can you communicate with key people in your network so that they can understand and support your change?

What other social situations do you anticipate being challenging? Make a list of the social challenges you are likely to face.

Inner blocks

What limiting beliefs or sabotaging behaviors may derail you? Do you have mixed feelings about making this change? Are there parts of you not fully on board? Perhaps you have people-pleasing tendencies that make it difficult to change your lifestyle. You may fear being different from others or fear that others won't approve of you. Maybe you tend to be too perfectionistic or hard on yourself. Or perhaps you are strongly attached to certain (non-vegan) foods and can't imagine changing what you eat.

One way to identify your mixed feelings and conflicts about change is to imagine having a *board meeting* with all the different "parts" of you. We all have a variety of "parts" with unique and differing qualities, characteristics, perspectives, and feelings.[6] Invite all the different aspects of yourself to express their feelings about your goal. You will have some parts of you that are excited and motivated, while others may have fears or concerns, or be resistant to change. Write down all the different thoughts and feelings that come up, without censoring or judging. Sometimes, it is enough to simply acknowledge and validate all the feelings, the positive ones, as well as the concerns, and nothing more needs to be done. There can be relief in just articulating all the different feelings and holding acceptance and compassion for them. At other times, you may need to offer inner reassurance or develop a plan to address and alleviate realistic concerns. Sometimes your conflicting feelings may bring wisdom, showing you where you need to grow or stretch, gather more support or information, or give yourself greater compassion and understanding.

Now that you have identified your practical, social, and inner barriers to change, let's explore how you can address these and get closer to your goals.

Set yourself up for success

To successfully start and sustain lifestyle changes, you need to create an inner and outer environment that supports you. Next, I discuss three key domains that can lay a strong foundation for your transition.

Seek information and resources

Knowledge is power—and it is essential for overcoming obstacles and reaching your goals. What information do you need to overcome the challenges you identified? What resources will help you? The Resources section at the back of this book has suggestions for books, websites, and documentaries where you can gain information, knowledge, and support.

If you want to move toward a vegan lifestyle, books such as *The 30-Day Vegan Challenge* by Colleen Patrick-Goudreau, *Main Street Vegan* by Victoria Moran, *The Vegan Way* by Jackie Day, *The Rebel Vegan Life* trilogy by Todd Sinclair, or *The Skinny on Eating Like You Give a Damn* by Stephanie Harter are great for providing valuable information and insights to get you started. In addition, the Resources section lists other books and resources focused on specific issues, such as nutrition, health, ethics, or the environment. For motivation and inspiration, watch documentaries such as *What the Health, Cowspiracy, Forks Over Knives, The Game Changers*, or *Peaceable Kingdom*. For ongoing encouragement and up-to-date information, find a plant-based or vegan podcast that you enjoy. Finally, see if there is a vegan advocacy or support group in your community. This can be invaluable for providing support, guidance, and information to nurture your transition.

Create a supportive environment

To create lasting change with less struggle, set up your home and social environment to support you. Often when we make dietary or lifestyle changes, we don't change our environment—and then we are surprised or disappointed when we lapse back into our old, familiar patterns. In my work with clients, and in the research on lifestyle change, the impact of one's environment on either supporting or derailing successful change cannot be overlooked.

For example, a closer look at the research on the Blue Zones finds that those who live in said Blue Zones are not necessarily more motivated or naturally healthy than the rest of us. It's just that their physical and social environment is set up to support healthier behaviors, such as eating more plants, moving more, living with purpose, and connecting with others.[7] Ideally, we would all have our own personal Blue Zone, with others who are engaged in the same healthy, compassionate, sustainable, plant-based lifestyle. However, for most of us, that is not the case, and we must be proactive in creating an environment that supports us.

First, take a look at the *practical* aspects of setting up your environment. Your research and information-gathering from the preceding sections will help you identify the specifics that you need to consider. It's important to remember that triggers in your environment can override your motivation, especially at times when you are tired or hungry or moody. If you are surrounded primarily by foods not on your eating plan, it will make change more difficult, especially in the early stages. That is why it's important to develop a strategy. This may include creating a weekly shopping list and planning your meals for the week; having plenty of fruits, veggies, and healthy plant-based snacks on hand; scheduling when you will prepare foods and cook; trying new vegan recipes; and removing the foods from your home that you will no longer be eating. If others in the household continue to eat these foods, you may want to work out an arrangement to have them stored separately, where they are less visible.

You will also want to develop a plan for eating out. For example, research online for restaurants that have vegan options or call restaurants ahead of time to determine how responsive they are to providing plant-based entrees. Search for appealing vegan dishes, whether you are eating out, shopping, or trying new recipes. Check cookbooks or search online to find vegan versions of your favorite foods and recipes. Try new foods as well; discover the delectable array of flavors, seasonings, and colorful ingredients in plant-based cooking.

Next, consider the *social* aspects of your environment. Be direct and clear with your loved ones, especially those with whom you spend time and eat meals. Share with them your reasons for making this lifestyle change, including the positives you hope to gain. If you are going vegan for ethical or environmental reasons, share a few of the factors motivating your decision. If you are moving toward a whole-food, plant-based lifestyle for better health, give a brief explanation of your reasons for this. It's usually best, at this point, not to overwhelm the other person with too much information, or endless facts and figures. Just share enough so that they can understand why this change is important to you, and perhaps be curious enough to want to learn more.

Ask your loved ones to be a support for you as you make this lifestyle change. Be specific about what support would be helpful. While you will want to set boundaries around your absolute needs (e.g., not permitting anyone to pressure you to eat animal foods or sabotage your goals), you may need to negotiate on *some* issues to find a mutually workable agreement (e.g., how to store or handle non-vegan foods in the house, if your partner or family members are not vegan). While you might wish that your loved ones would change their lifestyle along with you, this may or may not happen. If they are not immediately willing to go plant-based with you, enlist them to be a support for your change.[8]

Last, but not least, *connect with other vegans*, whether through local veg groups or online organizations. Spending time with others who are committed to the same lifestyle will help you stay motivated during times of discouragement, create a sense of connection, and give insights into how to handle common challenges. Revisit Chapter Six for more on the benefits of healthy support (and strategies for building support). For more help on dealing with social challenges, check out Chapter Ten and the Resources section.

Do your inner work

To empower your vegan/plant-based transition, it is important to also create a supportive *inner* environment. The following are some mindset shifts to increase your readiness and resilience:

- **Reconnect with your vision for change.** Revisit your intention and vision (that you identified earlier in this chapter) and the core values that underlie your goals. Whether your primary reason for change is for personal health, ethical reasons, animal compassion, spiritual alignment, and/or caring for the environment, review your WHY statement and action plan regularly to stay connected with your reasons for change and your plan for how to get there. This becomes your North Star, helping to realign you when life conspires to take you off track.

- **Continue to learn the benefits of plant-based living.** Those who have multiple motivating reasons for their vegan lifestyle (including those that extend beyond self to the greater good) are more likely to stay committed through tough times.[9] In addition, as you learn more about veganism and plant-based living, it will help you gain confidence that you can overcome any obstacles and challenges you may face.

- **Break through the trance of old habits.** Throughout the course of our lives, we acquire habits and preferences that become automatic. This is especially true when it comes to eating patterns. Adopting a vegan lifestyle causes us to confront many of our old patterns, habits, and assumptions. Whether it is your addiction to cheese, the societal message that you need animal protein, or ingrained cultural and family food traditions, shifting to a plant-based lifestyle will cause you to call these old patterns and beliefs into question. To overcome habits that hold you back, consider the following tools:

  o *Mindfulness*: Bring non-judgmental awareness to unhelpful patterns. Mindful awareness helps to break the trance of old habits.

  o *Mindset:* Remember WHY you are making this change and that you deserve to care for yourself and to honor your values.

  o *Information*: Learn the HOW of healthy plant-based eating so that you can undo misinformation, gain new insights, and discover solutions.

  o *Support*: Seek out others who have overcome these same problems, drawing from their wisdom and encouragement.

  o *Patience*: Remember that it takes time and practice to change old habits and develop new ones.

  o *Persistence*: Don't give up on yourself. Stay the course. It gets easier.

- **Let go of perfection or self-judgment.** It is normal to make mistakes or have setbacks when you are trying out new habits and lifestyle patterns. You may accidentally eat something you didn't plan to eat or give in to a friend's pressure. Have grace for yourself and use this as an opportunity to learn and grow. Those who are successful at lasting change learn to view setbacks and mistakes as learning opportunities. Instead of giving up when these happen, or beating up on yourself, see them for what they are—guidance for you to learn from so that you will be prepared next time. From my experience as a therapist and coach, I can't emphasize this enough. We all have setbacks. When they happen, be kind to yourself, let yourself feel your feelings (whether disappointment, discouragement, or frustration), then explore what you can learn, and move forward.

- **Celebrate the benefits of your new lifestyle.** You deserve to feel proud of your steps toward a plant-powered, vegan lifestyle. Give yourself positive messages as you make progress, whether you are learning new recipes or undoing old habits. In addition, pay attention to inner and outer positive changes that you experience. Many people notice physical benefits within days or weeks of adopting a plant-based diet. (Although, if you are making a big or sudden dietary change, be aware that there also could be a detox period; in this case, it is possible you may feel worse for a few days before feeling better). Other benefits may include emotional peace, greater confidence, authenticity, joy, or a sense of inner alignment. Also, celebrate the ways your lifestyle helps animals and the planet. Making this transition is not always easy, especially when others around you don't "get it," but remember that you are a leader and role model for positive change.

So, we've covered a lot here. Take your time with the questions and reflections just offered. Take one step at a time. As you take each step and gain confidence, the next steps will become clearer. Lean into your personal strengths and your past successes; remember your unique gifts and all that you have already overcome in your life.

The vegans that I interviewed each went through their own transition process, drawing on a wide variety of strategies for successfully embracing a vegan lifestyle. While their experiences differed, many embodied the principles described in this chapter. Next, I share the stories of Bobbi and Shannon. Bobbi's journey to becoming whole-food, plant-based (and later, an ethical vegan) unfolded over several years. Shannon, who was influenced by ethical concerns, shifted to a vegan diet virtually overnight, and veganized other aspects of her life (clothing, cosmetics, etc.) over time, as she learned more about each one. They each share the information and tactics that guided their vegan journey, as well as how their lives have changed as a result.

Bobbi's story

Bobbi Giudicelli is the author of *Freedom from a Toxic Relationship with Food*, which shares her journey to overcome her eating disorder and weight obsession, as well as tips and information to support others who struggle with these patterns. After years of disordered eating, the onset of chronic fatigue led her to take charge of her health. She ultimately embraced a whole-food, plant-based diet, and over time, also connected with her compassion for animals. She explained:

> My plant-based journey started about ten years ago, when my health was really struggling, as well as that of some of my family members. My sister had recently passed away from cancer, and as her primary caretaker, it was painful to watch her lose that battle. On top of that, around that same time, I watched my father's decline. I saw him go from an active man, who skied until he was eighty years old, to someone who was struggling to walk and who had progressive dementia for the last ten years of his life.
>
> At the same time, I noticed that my energy kept spiraling down, and I was struggling with "extreme fatigue," an actual disorder that far exceeds just "being tired." Daily activities, such as walking the length of my property, started to become insurmountable. All these things came together as the perfect trifecta (my father's, my sister's, and my own health) that became my wake-up call. I had always told myself that I ate pretty healthy, because I've been aware of and watched calories my whole life. I had some sense of what my caloric intake should be, and what I should eat as far as macronutrients, but I never took my understanding any further than that. My diet was probably not as bad as the standard American diet; I did eat a fair

amount of greens and veggies. But I also had plenty of unhealthy things. I was always managing calories, as opposed to managing nutrition.

After realizing I had hit bottom with my energy level, I started doing research into nutrition. I learned that all these health issues are tied to diet. It was like a major light bulb moment. First, I cleaned up my diet as far as processed foods and eliminated sugar and artificial sweeteners—especially diet soda. At first, I didn't try to give up animal products; like many people, I had concerns as to the impact on my everyday life, such as social engagements, ease of preparing meals, and so on. I thought, "It will be too hard. I'll feel deprived. It will be weird to go out to dinner with people." I had all these reasons not to consider veganism seriously. But as I started to eliminate processed foods, sugar, and then dairy, I realized this isn't so hard. Not only is it not hard, but I also feel so much better! Once I started making changes, it was easy. I made it easy and rewarding. Gradually, I eliminated other animal-based foods, the last ones being fish and eggs. Now, I look at foods that I thought I couldn't live without, and I wouldn't even think to eat them. I just wouldn't. I can't even imagine going back in any way. I've been 100 percent vegan and whole foods plant-based for over six years now.

Since changing my diet, I feel more energetic. I don't know exactly when the improvement started, whether it was when I eliminated processed food, or when I eliminated all animal products. I just know that I have much more energy than I had ten, twenty, even thirty years ago. I also found out that I was sensitive to gluten, and my digestion is much better since stopping that. Now, I feel balanced. I feel cleansed. I've been an athlete my whole life and have had many orthopedic surgeries; I used to be constantly inflamed and feel tremendous pain in many of my joints. Now, I have minimal to no inflammation in my body. I learned in my research that animal products are inflammatory. I play pickleball now with people my age and up to twenty years younger than I am; they've got knee braces, back braces, and arm braces on and they're hobbling around, while I'm moving around as well as I did when I was thirty, more than three decades ago.

The biggest benefit by far, however, is my emotional health. For many years, my emotional health was impacted by what I had been eating, how much I had been eating, and my weight. I had very high highs and very low lows. With the lows came a lack of patience, great agitation, and often a feeling of malaise. I can honestly say, in retrospect, that my spouse wasn't sure which version of me would walk in the door at the end of the day. Since adopting a vegan lifestyle, I experience much improved mental clarity and increased emotional stability. Along with that came added joy, gratitude, and overall satisfaction with my life, marriage, and friendships.

I am somebody who has a complete conviction that our purpose on this planet is to be of service. Every business that I've been a part of has had a social commitment. When I really woke up and embraced a full vegan lifestyle, that felt good, like I was doing something worthwhile. Since changing the way I eat, I can honestly tell you, I experience joy, gratification, and satisfaction on a regular basis. I've always been a passionate person. But now it's side by side with the joy that I experience. I've always been an animal lover. So many good things have come from my relationships with different animals. I wonder, how could I not have made that connection [with what I ate]? When I was writing my book, I included a section about veganism; I realized that I wanted to draw a line in the sand and say, "This is how I live, and here is why."

Shannon's story

Shannon is a relatively new vegan, who made her transition about a year before our interview. When I asked what led her to go vegan, she said:

It was my love of Harry Potter. I listened to a Harry Potter podcast, and they interviewed actress Evanna Lynch (who played Luna Lovegood). That led me to listen to her *Chickpeeps* podcast. And listening to that informed me of all the stuff that goes on with animals. I had always turned a blind eye before. That day, I came home and told my husband, "We're gonna have to figure something out. Because I think I need to go vegan. I don't think I can see any other way."

My transition was pretty much overnight. I thought I would finish up whatever cheese or meat was in the house, and then just not buy it again. But when I tried to eat cheese again, I couldn't bring myself to do it. My husband isn't vegan, so he finished up that stuff. I've been slower with transitioning my clothing and cosmetics, I just had no idea how to go about it at first. I've been learning and slowly working my way into it.

Shannon said that her husband, although not vegan himself, has been supportive. "He told me if I could make a vegan quiche that he liked, he would be willing to eat vegan meals for dinner. He ended up liking my plant-based meals better than he liked my cooking before." Shannon started by doing Google searches for vegan versions of recipes and trying them out. She also found cookbooks she likes; a current favorite is *PlantYou* by Carleigh Bodrug.

> I'm a super visual learner. This cookbook literally shows you a picture of each ingredient, and what the dish looks like when it's completed. The recipes and instructions are doable and not too complicated. I'm not a chef, so it's great that she uses ingredients that are easy to find at the store.

Shannon acknowledged some rough spots during her first holidays as a vegan:

> Mom asked me, "Well, what about grandma's pumpkin pie? What about the holidays?" My first Thanksgiving as a vegan was tough, because no one made anything that was vegan. I still had plenty to eat, but only because I brought five dishes that I made. Christmas with my family was interesting. My dad is gluten-free, so I was trying to make things vegan and gluten-free. My mom brought the turkey in a crockpot, so I didn't have to stare at a turkey the whole time. I did all the side dishes, and I veganized them all. And my dad, surprisingly, said they were really good. However, the pumpkin pie wasn't quite the same texture as they were used to. I told my mom, "It's still a work in progress."
>
> My mom initially thought it was just a phase. I think now that it's been about a year, she's realizing, "Oh, maybe this isn't a phase." And she's realized that she ends up having problems when she eats a lot of dairy products, so, she's started eating less dairy. And then, I made a kale salad recipe the other day. At first, she said she didn't like kale, but she tried it and said, "Oh, this is good. Can you send me the recipe?"
>
> My inner growth started when I made a New Year's resolution to learn how to say "No" a couple of years ago. In a way, that led to my journey to becoming vegan. I left my previous work as a teacher, because I was a natural introvert, and I was so stressed that I was coping with emotional eating and overeating. I've struggled with

my weight my whole life, but I was gaining even more weight and stopping for takeout on the way home because I was too tired to make dinner. After that, I found a new job where I'm happy. And ever since becoming vegan, I found that my attitude toward myself improved. I found it easier to feel good about myself because I was not putting junk into my body. After I went vegan, it was easier to talk more positively to myself. And on top of that, I've been able to lose twenty-five pounds so far.

I'm no longer ashamed to be different. I've come to the realization that I am a vegan who also has a strong faith in God; I've realized I'm a unique person. It's helped my spirituality grow more. It's this whole string of events and people that led me on this path. And looking back on it, I can see the work of God in my life. I had a lot of negative self-talk and low self-esteem that carried through much of my life. I also was a people-pleaser. I tried to work on it prior to becoming vegan, but when I tried to change to more positive self-talk, I didn't necessarily believe it. When I became vegan, it was just more natural. I was like, "Whoa, this is weird. I haven't been talking negatively to myself." I now have more of a calm confidence in myself and my choices. It feels like I'm finally becoming the person who God wanted me to be.

Shannon and Bobbi's stories showcase how the transition to a plant-based, vegan lifestyle can be, for many, a journey of discovery that propels physical healing along with psychological and spiritual growth. Their journeys also highlight the importance of being open to adopting a new mindset and learning to adapt to situations in new ways. For many vegans, the biggest challenges, especially early on, are the emotional and social challenges of living in a not-yet-vegan world. The next chapter offers suggestions for not only managing these challenges but also thriving.

CHAPTER 10

THRIVING EMOTIONALLY AND SOCIALLY WITH A VEGAN LIFESTYLE

"For many vegans, the decision to stop consuming animals is one of the most empowering choices of their lives. And yet this decision often comes at a price—the disruption of relationships . . . Fortunately, relationship breakdown is not inevitable, nor is it irreversible. In fact, becoming vegan is an opportunity to strengthen connections and improve the health of relationships."

—**Melanie Joy**, Ph.D. in *Beyond Beliefs* [1]

"Veganism is not a limitation in any way. It's an expansion of your love, your commitment to nonviolence, and your belief in justice for all."

—**Gary Francione**, law professor, author, and animal rights activist

The unique social and emotional landscape for vegans

As discussed in Chapter Nine, lifestyle change is often a process that involves learning new information, developing new skills, and changing mindsets and habits. While change in and of itself can be difficult, becoming vegan entails its own unique challenges. As Melanie Joy points out in the preceding quote, and as showcased throughout this book, becoming vegan can be one of the most empowering decisions we make. And yet, for a variety of reasons, in becoming vegan we may face social opposition, disbelief, judgment, or criticism that can catch us off guard. We may also experience difficult emotions, such as grief, sadness, or anger, when we learn about the widespread cruelty to animals in many industries and realize the devastating consequences of animal agriculture.

In this chapter, I discuss some of the social challenges and emotional impacts that vegans may face. Subsequently, I offer tools to help navigate these challenges, to empower yourself to thrive.

Social challenges

Handling social situations can be among the biggest hurdles for those adopting a vegan lifestyle. We bond with others through shared meals and traditions around food; when these familiar traditions are disrupted by our diet and lifestyle changes (and all the new awarenesses that accompany this), we may experience pushback from those in our social circle. This pushback can lead us to feel isolated or disconnected, particularly if others criticize, mock, or disregard our values. My survey respondents reported that their most common social stressors included lack of vegan options at social events, lack of support, and negative reactions regarding their veganism. Some vegans reported that they had been ridiculed or verbally attacked for their vegan choices or had been excluded from a social gathering due to being vegan. Many expressed anxiety or stress about attending social events where animal foods were present.

Why the negative reactions from those in our social network to our decision to become vegan? To be clear, not everyone reports problematic experiences, and hopefully, as veganism and plant-based living become more widespread, these types of problems will be much less common. However, at the present time, those who courageously embrace a vegan lifestyle are still early adopters, part of a small percentage of the global population who have made the decision to eliminate animal products in the name of compassion, ethics, health, and the well-being of the planet. As those on the forefront of emerging social change, we are likely to experience negative responses from others, and it is helpful to gain understanding about the factors that contribute.

Once we realize the detrimental effects of animal agriculture and other exploitative industries, in terms of cruelty to animals, harm to human health, and destruction of the planet, we often wonder why others around us don't also see this. We may urgently try to tell them what we've learned, only to be dismissed, silenced, ridiculed, or ignored. How can this be? How can other compassionate, rational people dismiss the evidence we are sharing?

Like many vegans, I have wrestled with this question. I have had to remind myself that my own awakening did not start until I was forty, and even then, it took several years to embrace a vegan lifestyle. Many vegans change much more quickly than I did. It seems that it is becoming more common to make the change "overnight," since information is more readily available, and veganism is becoming more mainstream. Even so, as vegans, we discover quickly that not everyone around us "wakes up" just because we did, or is willing to change in the same way or timeframe.

There are many social, cultural, and psychological factors that play into why people may resist veganism. For example, as discussed in Chapter Two, we are raised to believe it is natural and healthy to eat certain animals. This social conditioning is deeply ingrained and is imperceptible to us. It is part of the water we have always swam in. As a result, we are not receptive to new insights and ways of being. In addition, we develop (often unconscious) emotional ties to certain foods that have been part of family upbringing and traditions. This, in turn, drives our eating behavior and our reluctance to make changes. On top of this, our fear of being different, being rejected or excluded, or standing out can block us from eating differently than those in our social circle. We are each unique in the degree to which these social and psychological factors influence us and hold us back from openness to learning about veganism.

It's also important to remember that many corporate interests are invested in obscuring the cruelty, exploitation, and suffering caused to animals in agriculture and other industries, so that the average person does not see or even think about this. Conflicting messages and misinformation from the media and other authorities add to the collective confusion and apathy surrounding these issues. Many vegans experience distress when they become aware of the extensive harms of exploitative industries, especially as they realize that they have been misled by societal authorities that they trusted.

When you consider these complex social, cultural, historical, economic, and psychological factors and interests that play into our norms around eating animals, and how embedded these norms still are, it's not surprising that vegans may experience social repercussions when they choose to no longer participate in this system. Many of us who become vegan find that when we share our perspectives, our reasons for being vegan, or simply say that we are vegan, non-vegans may react defensively. Vegans' social challenges are sometimes intensified because we may not have the communication skills needed to effectively express ourselves amidst all these complexities—and instead may communicate in ways that further distance or alienate ourselves from others.

Emotional challenges

Because our social relationships are central to our well-being and ability to thrive, when we experience conflict, disconnection, or disruption in our relationships, this shakes us emotionally and can contribute to feelings of loneliness, isolation, sadness, anger, or frustration. Thus, learning to navigate social challenges, build healthy support, and communicate more effectively are foundational to emotionally thriving as a vegan, as well as thriving as a human being in general.

In addition to these social-emotional challenges, vegans may experience varying levels of emotional distress upon learning about the cruelty to animals and the planetary destruction caused by animal agriculture and other industries. Many of my survey respondents said that they have experienced sadness, grief, and anger along their vegan journey. Some acknowledged that they have experienced despair or hopelessness about ongoing animal suffering and/or environmental degradation. A smaller number of participants had at some point experienced more severe emotional distress, such as depression, anxiety, or traumatic stress symptoms.

These emotions are compounded by negative reactions from others. We assume that others will be shocked, as we were, by this information about animal cruelty, human health, and/or the environment. Many of us feel devastated, unsupported, or frustrated when others dismiss or reject what we are sharing. It's emotionally distressing to learn of atrocities such as those enacted upon animals, and even more difficult to carry this distress alone. It is natural to experience grief and disillusionment under these circumstances—even more so for those on the front lines of animal advocacy, who regularly witness and protest violence and cruelty toward animals.

Vegan psychologist Clare Mann created the term *Vystopia* to describe the existential angst that many vegans experience upon learning about the systematized abuse and exploitation of animals; exploitation that is societally supported (whether knowingly or not) through our daily purchases and food choices. Mann, who is also a psychotherapist, animal rights advocate, international speaker, and author of the book *Vystopia: The Anguish of Being Vegan in a Non-Vegan World*, found that many vegans and animal rights activists describe similar emotional reactions and symptoms. These can include complicated grief, anxiety, despair, emotional anguish, guilt at not being able to do enough to help animals, alienation from others, post-traumatic stress disorder symptoms, and, in some cases, depression or suicidal thoughts. She contends that this existential anguish is not a sign of pathology; rather, it is an understandable response to "the burden of knowing" that vegans experience when they learn of the extensive harm and violence done to animals.[2] She tells us, "People *should* be outraged and pained when they discover the enormous industrial cover-up in society and complacency people have with this systemized cruelty."[3]

Some vegans who witness significant violence or cruelty to animals (whether through front-line animal activism or watching disturbing video footage) may experience symptoms of traumatic stress. Trauma is the internal wound (and resulting symptoms) that we may experience in response to hurtful or violent events. Dr. Gabor Maté, a physician, author, and renowned expert in addictions and stress, describes trauma as a "psychic injury, lodged in our nervous system, mind, and body, lasting long past the originating incident(s), triggerable at any moment." He explains that trauma is not the devastating events themselves, but rather the inner scarring that forms in response to these events, which affects our emotions, world view, beliefs, narratives, and resulting coping mechanisms. Trauma exists on a continuum, ranging from milder, less intense responses to more severe forms that impact our daily functioning.[4]

You have most likely heard of *post-traumatic stress disorder* (PTSD), which may affect those who experience a traumatic event such as assault, abuse, injury, combat, or threat of harm or death. Those who *indirectly* experience trauma (e.g., first responders, activists, or others who witness or are exposed to violence toward others) also may be at risk for PTSD. (Note: this indirect traumatization has also been called *secondary traumatic stress* or *vicarious trauma*). PTSD symptoms include intrusive thoughts and images of distressing or violent scenes, heightened physiological reactivity, negative thoughts and feelings related to traumatic events, sleep difficulties, anxiety, and trouble concentrating. Those diagnosed with PTSD experience these symptoms with a frequency, intensity, and duration that cause disruptions in daily functioning.[5] Vegans and activists with indirect traumatization from witnessing violence toward others may experience additional challenges, such as feeling overly responsible for fixing the problem(s), along with a sense of guilt that they are not able to do enough. They also may tend to neglect their own needs, believing that they are less important in comparison with those who have been harmed.[6]

For those who may be experiencing traumatic stress and/or Vystopia symptoms, learning that these are understandable responses to violence, harm, and oppression can bring tremendous relief and empowerment. We can gain skills to cope and to transform emotional distress into empowered and resourceful action. With our new awareness, we can discern when we would benefit from additional help and/or professional treatment to support our healing journey. The remainder of this chapter addresses skills, mindsets, and resources for empowered coping and thriving.

Tools to empower yourself to thrive

I want to reiterate that vegans are a diverse group of people who have varied experiences, and the same holds true with their emotional and social experiences. Some vegans who responded to my survey expressed that they didn't have significant emotional or social challenges, and/or that they learned to work through any challenges they initially experienced. Some, however, struggled to come to terms with the extensive harm to animals, and society's complacency surrounding this. For example, one survey respondent said, "My view of the world and mankind is now shattered."

Many participants, while acknowledging distress about the harmful effects of animal agriculture, said that becoming vegan uplifted them and brought empowerment and freedom. As expressed by Jane Velez-Mitchell, creator of UnchainedTV, "While upset and even angry and sad about unnecessary animal suffering, we [vegans] are also happy, joyous, and free." Another research participant commented, "Becoming vegan was the best decision I have made . . . I still feel sad and angry about this injustice. At the same time, there is nothing that makes me feel happier and more alive than my choice to be vegan." Many lamented that their primary regret was that they did not become vegan sooner.

The vast majority of research participants found ways to cope with their challenges and rise above them, to become more resilient, fulfilled, and impactful. Next, I describe nine tools to support you in emotionally thriving on your vegan journey. These tips are drawn from the responses of my survey participants, who shared the mindsets, skills, and approaches they found most helpful for coping and thriving. In addition, these tools incorporate my experience as a therapist and coach, as well as the wisdom of vegan experts who teach and write on this topic.[7]

1. The power of your convictions

In *Man's Search for Meaning*, Victor Frankl quotes Nietzsche: "He who has a WHY to live for can bear almost any HOW." Frankl argued that those who have a sense of purpose and a vision for the future (a strong WHY) are more likely to be resilient, even amid terrible circumstances and difficulties. He found this to be true for those living in the horrific conditions of the concentration camps, as well as for those facing more typical life challenges.[8]

The power of being driven by inner convictions (a strong WHY) was expressed by my survey respondents as well. When I asked participants what helped them cope with any challenges associated with being vegan, many responded with some variation of the following:

- "I am certain I am on the right path and doing my part."
- "I know I am doing the right thing."

- "Knowing that what I am doing is the compassionate and loving thing to do."
- "I am resolute and committed to my values."
- "Staying true to my convictions."
- "Reminding myself that I am living the most cruelty-free lifestyle that I can."
- "I know that what I am doing is bigger than me and a little discomfort is worth it."
- "Staying true to my inner conscience."
- "Knowing I am saving animals' lives and living the most peaceful way."

Veganism is an embodiment of values such as compassion, peace, justice, love, health, and reverence for life. When we realize that we can make a difference for animals' lives, our own health, and the planet through our daily food choices, it becomes easier to stay the course despite any challenges or difficulties. In fact, we become *committed* to overcoming these obstacles. Our strong WHY makes us determined to figure out the HOW.

My research respondents' strong convictions helped them view the challenges of a vegan lifestyle as something they could (and were determined to) cope with and overcome. In addition, their convictions served to remind them that, in becoming vegan, they were doing something to make a positive difference. This gave them a measure of hope, a sense that they were doing their part to create a kinder, more peaceful world. Living by their convictions often gave a sense of purpose, fulfillment, and joy, even in the midst of difficulties.

For many, this strong sense of conviction comes quickly upon learning about animal exploitation and cruelty. For others, conviction comes from a determination to heal from disease. However, because of our societal conditioning and the pervasiveness of animal products in our culture, we may need to remind ourselves of the reasons for our vegan choice from time to time, especially early in our vegan journey. Remembering our reasons for choosing a vegan lifestyle, and continuing to add to these reasons, helps us remain intentional about our lifestyle choices, rather than falling back into the trance of familiar, socially prevalent patterns.

When I decided to become vegan, I had already been vegetarian for several years, and was fully committed to not eating meat. The mere thought of it brought up distressing, vivid images of how farmed animals were raised and slaughtered. However, discontinuing dairy was more difficult for me; it was so ubiquitous and often invisible in many foods. Early on, I felt anxiety about declining (non-vegan) birthday cake at a family gathering. I didn't want to make a scene at what was supposed to be a celebratory occasion. I was still processing what I was discovering about the dairy and egg industries, and I alternated between feeling distraught and overwhelmed to just wanting to go along with the social flow and not think about it. It was after I did more reading and emotionally connected with the horrific conditions for dairy cows and egg-laying hens that I became determined to figure out how to speak up and honor my values. At that point, my convictions were strong enough that I knew it was worth it to overcome any social difficulties or inconveniences.

When asked, "What has helped you cope with any challenges associated with being vegan?" many respondents reported a similar process of connecting with their convictions, as shown in the survey responses here:

> "I check back often with my core beliefs. I know I don't want to support violence and cruelty toward animals, or anyone for that matter, including myself. I feel as if I have become more of an adult, a person settled in truth."

> "Just being solid and confident that this is the right, moral, ethical, and healthy thing to do. Knowing there is not a single 'contraindication' to being vegan."

> "I've learned to be okay with being different, knowing I am doing the right thing."

> "Knowing without a doubt that I made the right decision, and that no obstacle would prevent me from being true to myself. I've found power in saying no and strength in doing the right thing."

2. Advance your knowledge

I've mentioned the value of continued learning throughout this book, but it bears repeating. Those who thrive as vegans are often those who continue to educate themselves on relevant issues. This includes learning about the ethical, environmental, health, and other benefits of a vegan lifestyle; how to respond to others' questions about vegan issues; handling social situations; healthy communication skills; and the psychology of food choices.

This doesn't mean you have to be an expert on all things vegan. However, staying informed helps you to thrive in a number of ways:

- It keeps you inspired about your motivations for being vegan.
- It helps you to successfully navigate the vegan landscape, from practical challenges, to learning the basics of plant-based nutrition, to handling social pressures.
- It can help you become a better communicator and advocate for vegan living.
- It provides encouraging role models for thriving as a vegan.
- It can nurture hope, empowerment, and resilience.

With any lifestyle change, we need support and information to help us succeed. With a vegan lifestyle, this is even more essential. We need to learn from others who have handled the same situations and share the same values. This gives us confidence to walk on new terrain. It also gives us wisdom to respond to other people's questions and not be derailed by negative comments. It reminds us of all the reasons we decided to take the vegan path, and the many benefits to us, animals, and the world that result.

Seek out the information that inspires and supports you. You can learn in whatever ways work best for you. You may enjoy books, audiobooks, documentaries, podcasts, articles, informative websites, presentations, networking groups, and/or courses on vegan issues or plant-based living. Many survey respondents indicated that continued learning has helped them to thrive on their vegan journey, as shared here:

"It's helped me to gain more knowledge. I've learned about positive ways to be a vegan advocate from an excellent workshop by Dr. Melanie Joy. I now realize that people will often attack or feel defensive because, deep down, they know that what they are doing is wrong. I was a meat-eater once, although a very long time ago, and now recognize that this is carnism at play."

"[What has helped is] educating myself on the WHYs. It's not up to me to convince or change others, but I can inspire with my deep conviction and the consequences of my food choices on my own health."

> "I listen to YouTube talks by plant-based doctors and others following this lifestyle. I read continuously about health and the WFPB lifestyle."

3. Find your tribe

In Chapter Six "The Power of True Connection" I discussed that one of the joys of becoming vegan is connecting with a like-minded and like-hearted tribe. We are naturally uplifted and fulfilled when we connect with others who share our values, perspectives, concerns, and commitment. And, because our world's dominant ideology is still carnistic (i.e., holding the belief that it is appropriate and necessary to eat certain animals),[9] we need the support of others who share our awareness and convictions. This helps to not only sustain a vegan lifestyle, but also to increase fulfillment, well-being, and flourishing. Our vegan friends can also share their insights on how they have handled and overcome challenges along the way.

When I asked survey respondents what helps them to cope with challenges, support from other vegans came up frequently, whether through friendships, networking groups, plant-based support groups, volunteering, or involvement in a vegan organization. The responses that follow highlight the value of kindred vegan support.

> "I feel a deep level of connection when I talk to other vegans. We already share a similar foundation. I don't have to explain my concern for animals, they already get it. I don't have to worry I will be judged or misunderstood."

> "When I'm struggling, I talk things over with my dear vegan friend."

> "I create vegan community wherever and whenever I can, as well as spiritual community with those who have similar concerns, but may not be vegan (yet)."

> "I connect with online communities, listen to vegan podcasts, and attend Veg Fests."

4. Be proactive when it comes to social events and eating out

As vegans, we quickly learn the importance of planning ahead. It is easier to be prepared in our own homes, where we can develop routines such as meal planning, grocery shopping, scheduled cooking time, and stocking our pantry and fridge with plant-based staples and snacks. However, we may be thrown off-guard at social events or when traveling, when we discover, to our dismay, that there are no vegan/plant-based options available.

This happened to me more than once before I learned that I needed to be proactive if I wanted to enjoy non-vegan social events and not be hungry. Here are some suggestions to proactively approach these situations:

- For social events, talk to the host or hostess ahead of time. Let them know you are vegan, what you eat and don't eat, and ask if they would be okay with you bringing a vegan dish to share, and/or if they are comfortable providing something vegan.

- For potlucks or holiday meals, bring delectable food to share. Not only will you ensure that you have something to eat, but you also offer the opportunity for others to experience how appealing plant-based cuisine can be.

- When eating out, use the Happy Cow app[10] or other online sites to find vegan and veg-friendly restaurants. If you are going to a restaurant that doesn't have obvious vegan options, it helps to call ahead or talk with a staff member to see what options are available. Some restaurants have a separate vegan menu that is only handed out if someone asks. If there are no vegan options, ask for adjustments to existing menu items to make them vegan.

- When there is no opportunity to check ahead about vegan options, you may want to eat some food ahead of time or bring snacks, just to be on the safe side.

- For travel, it is helpful to bring plenty of vegan snacks and staples.

- Assume that others (hosts, restaurant owners and staff, etc.) want to support you. While you may encounter those unwilling to offer vegan options, most often, your host wants you to have a positive experience. However, don't assume they know how to support you; the prevailing social conditioning can create a blind spot around what veganism means. Be direct and specific about your needs.

At first, I was somewhat resistant to being proactive. After all, I'd lived my whole life eating what everyone else did, so it had never been necessary before. However, when I reconnected with my reasons for choosing a vegan lifestyle, and reminded myself I was taking the road less traveled, I realized it was worth it to develop new skills to navigate this road successfully. The importance of proactive planning also frequently came up in the responses of my survey participants:

> "I'm proactive about getting my needs met. I call ahead to restaurants to see if I need to eat a small meal before I go out should menu items not meet my nutritional needs. I remind others that I respect their right to make food choices according to their beliefs and I ask others to do the same."

> "If I'm the 'odd' one out, I just go prepared with my own food and see it as an opportunity to inspire others. If I'm invited to events like horse races, I would just decline and politely say why, and hope I plant some seeds along the way."

> "I bring my own food, or fill up ahead of time, when attending events with few or no vegan options. I never feel pressured to eat animal products and never would even if someone felt insulted that I didn't eat their food. When I go to a restaurant with non-vegan friends, I eat vegan options, or simply order steamed veggies with pasta or a salad."

5. Become a better communicator

Many of these tools for thriving rest on our ability to be effective communicators. This is not an ability we are necessarily born with; most of us need to work to develop our communication skills. Whether it is speaking up with the host of a social event, the wait staff at a restaurant, your mother or mother-in-law, your partner, your boss, or the person at the gym who makes an obnoxious comment about your vegan T-shirt, you need skills to communicate successfully.

There is an art to effective and generative communication. With some people and situations, communication flows smoothly and naturally, and we don't have to give it a lot of thought. However, for highly stressful or triggering situations, we will likely need to strengthen our skills for handling these. When a relationship conflict keeps recurring (for example, your mom says she will provide a vegan option for you, but then repeatedly "forgets"), it can be helpful to take a time-out to pause and clarify your intentions and desires for the situation. You may want to calm yourself and connect with your Wise Brain (the part of your brain that holds emotional intelligence) before engaging in a potentially emotionally charged conversation. The book *Crucial Conversations: Tools for Talking When the Stakes Are High* suggests asking yourself questions such as: "What do I really want for myself, for the other person, and for the relationship? And how would I behave if I really wanted those results?" In other words, what is the best way to express myself to create the outcome I truly desire?[11]

In general, an *assertive communication* approach (rather than being overly passive, aggressive, or passive-aggressive) is most effective for working through conflicts, increasing mutual understanding, and/or requesting change. Assertive communication entails expressing your feelings and needs clearly and directly, in a way that is respectful of the other person (as well as yourself). When you communicate assertively, you are honest about what you feel, where you stand, and what you would like to see happen, and at the same time, do this in a way that honors the dignity of the other person.[12]

Passive communication, in contrast, is when we don't speak up at all, or dance around the issues, rather than be clear and direct. Often this occurs when we are trying to please others or avoid conflict. In this approach, we undermine or minimize our own needs and wishes.

Aggressive communication comes across as hostile, contemptuous, or threatening. It can range from an angry tone of voice, to name-calling, to verbal abuse, to physical violence. While aggressive communication may have its place (for example, if responding to a direct threat or danger), in general, it is not an effective communication approach. Those on the receiving end of aggression tend to feel threatened, which often triggers a fight-or-flight response. This triggered state may lead the other person to respond back with anger or aggression (fight), or to withdraw, avoid, or escape (flight). *Passive-aggressive behavior* is a more subtle form of aggression, which can include sarcasm, ridicule, or undermining behaviors.

The authors of *Crucial Conversations* studied the approaches utilized by effective communicators and leaders. They found that effective communicators were neither passive or aggressive, but rather took responsibility for addressing problems and conflicts head-on and did so in ways that led to mutual safety, meaningful dialogue, finding common ground, and often uncovering new, creative solutions.[13] If this feels like a tall order, you are not alone in finding this to be difficult. When we feel triggered by others, we tend to go into fight-or-flight mode, and it is hard to think clearly how to respond.

Start by clarifying your intentions and desires regarding any problematic social situations or interpersonal conflicts you are facing. What do you hope to create—for yourself, for the other(s) involved, and for the larger picture? This reflection reconnects you with your deeper wishes, rather than being reactive. Once you have identified what you truly want for the relationship and/or situation, you can then determine what you need to move forward. Maybe you are ready to have that tough conversation, or maybe you first need to talk it through with an understanding friend or read a book that improves your communication literacy.[14]

Developing communication skills occurs over time and with practice. While being vegan in a not-yet-vegan world can be a source of conflict, it can also be an opportunity to strengthen our communication and relational skills, as we learn how to work through differences. We may, over time, develop empathy for those who are at different places on their journey and learn to communicate in ways that connect and inspire, rather than separate. We discover that we can create healthy relationships that allow us (and others) the space to be our full selves, as expressed by my survey respondents:

> "I've learned to speak up and express myself in non-defensive and non-judgmental ways."

> "I needed to build my self-esteem to know that I was deserving of respect for my beliefs, deserving of being served a meal I can eat, as my colleagues were. And from this self-esteem came greater assertiveness."

> "While I've had times of upset or hurt at someone's comments, it's always an opportunity for growth, for me to learn how to better respond, to be a better communicator."

"I'm vocal about my needs and boundaries. I give family members the benefit of the doubt and don't assume they will "get it" according to my timeline. I find other areas of common ground with non-vegan friends and family. I continue to educate myself and help educate others."

6. Include yourself in your circle of care

Many vegans hold deep compassion for non-human animals. What we may forget is that we too are animals, sentient beings who have physical, emotional, mental, and spiritual needs. When we extend kindness and care for *all beings*, it's important to include ourselves in the equation. The vegans that I surveyed repeatedly emphasized the value of daily self-care practices to help cope and to thrive. This included healthy plant-based nutrition, exercise, meditation, spiritual practices, time in nature, time with companion animals, and visiting sanctuaries. Alongside these practices was developing greater self-compassion and self-love. Many came to realize that in order to be the change they wanted to see in the world, they needed to also treat themselves as deserving of self-kindness. Respondents shared practices that helped them cope and stay grounded. For example:

- "I focus on the things I can control. I try not to let the things that are beyond my sphere of influence make me feel anxious or depressed."
- "I practice mindfulness every day, and this helps greatly."
- "I cope through spiritual practices, like prayer and meditation."
- "I take long walks in the woods, I cry when I need to, write in my diary, and talk with other vegans."
- "I have started meditating and connecting to nature."
- "I try to extend compassion to myself and other humans, since I already have compassion for most other species."

7. Manage empathic distress

When we learn about the horrific conditions for farmed animals, or witness videos of the slaughter process, this can leave a deep impact on us emotionally. As discussed in Chapter Three "Expand Your Circle of Compassion," our compassion and desire to alleviate suffering is an admirable and healthy part of our humanity. And yet, repeatedly witnessing horrifying, violent scenes, especially if we feel helpless or powerless, may leave us vulnerable to empathic distress and/or traumatic stress. Those who courageously work in direct activism on behalf of animals may face even greater exposure to traumatic images. Compassionate advocates may believe that their own emotional difficulties are insignificant in comparison to what the animals are facing, and that all attention should go to the animals.

However, to draw on a commonly used analogy: we need to put on our own oxygen masks first, in order to be of true help. It is difficult to be a sustainable vegan advocate or to bring about systemic change if we ourselves are not doing well emotionally or physically. As expressed by one research respondent, "I realized that being stuck in depression or anger won't help the animals." To thrive as a vegan, and to have greater impact for causes we care about, we need to develop emotional self-care skills. The following are some suggestions:

- **Limit your exposure to disturbing images, videos, and social media posts.** Some vegans feel they need to watch these continually, to be motivated on behalf of the animals. While it may be helpful (and important) to view these on occasion, for many of us, repeated exposure to traumatic images is too much for our nervous systems to handle well. Once you have made the connection about animal exploitation and suffering, it is usually not necessary to revisit this footage, unless it's an essential part of your work as an activist. As expressed by one survey respondent: "I no longer watch films or undercover footage depicting animal cruelty. For a while, I needed reminders of why I became vegan, but that is no longer the case, and I can't stomach the images anymore."

- **Learn skills to process and regulate your emotions.** It's normal to feel sad, angry, and/or distressed about exploitation and suffering. Learning how to process your emotions, and to let them move through you, is essential so that emotions don't get "stuck." As one vegan explained: "I've learned to give myself room to have the tough feelings and work through them." There are a variety of approaches to help, many of which center on the concept of mindfulness. Mindfulness teaches us to witness and acknowledge our thoughts and emotions, notice where they are held in the body, and detach from our identification with them. Mindfulness has been shown to calm the nervous system and allows us to handle stressors with less overwhelm. Mindfulness is also key for holding compassion in ways that empower us and lessen the risk of empathic overwhelm and burnout.[15]

- **Take extra care if you are an empath or a highly sensitive person.** If you seem to be more sensitive than others around you, you may have a nervous system that is wired for greater empathy and/or sensitivity. Those who are highly empathic or sensitive are often very conscientious and committed to helping others. Yet, this neurological sensitivity may lead to overwhelm in situations that are disturbing or overstimulating, especially if you don't have the skills to manage this. If this sounds like you, it can be very helpful to empower yourself with strategies, knowledge, and resources made for highly sensitive, empathic people.[16]

- **Know when to seek help.** If you experience severe symptoms of traumatic stress (described earlier in this chapter), empathic overwhelm, and/or other emotional symptoms that are disrupting your life, consider seeking support from a therapist or professional who is well-versed in vegan issues, trauma, and/or Vystopia. The support of a trained professional who not only understands your feelings and concerns, but also offers tools for coping, can make a world of difference.[17]

8. Make a positive impact

Joan Baez, the songwriter and activist, is noted for saying, "Action is the antidote to despair." Many of the vegans I surveyed shared this philosophy. They found that being actively involved in a cause that matters to them makes all the difference in their own well-being and gives a sense of hope and purpose. Whatever the cause that most speaks to you, whether human health, mental health, animal protection, climate healing, world hunger, injustice or oppression, or any other issue, taking positive action can move you from powerless to empowered. This might be a good time to revisit

Chapter Four "Connect with Deeper Meaning and Purpose" to discover what is calling you. My survey respondents shared the benefits of making a meaningful contribution:

> "Activism is the antidote to despair and hopelessness. Instead of letting those negative feelings bring me down, I channel them into determination to change something, make something a little better in the world."

> "To cope with hopelessness, I try to channel every part of my life into alleviating animal suffering, whether that's fostering cats, investing in vegan startups, writing about veganism and health, or donating to animal rights causes."

> "I work every day to make the world better for animals and to wake people up to the horrors and cruelty of factory farming, its impact on their health and on habitat destruction, wildlife extinction, human world hunger, human disease, and especially climate change. I also know that being sad and depressed does not help animals. As long as I do something to help each day, I give myself permission to be happy."

9. Build hope for a better world

Finally, to thrive emotionally, we need to nurture hope. As noted earlier, one way to strengthen hope is to work with others toward a cause that you are passionate about—and to recognize that you are making a positive difference. In addition, you can nurture hope by bringing your awareness to the positives that are happening around you. You may have heard the phrase: "What you focus on expands." When we *only* notice the pain and injustice in the world, it keeps us stuck in a negative place. When we intentionally notice the good that is happening, it allows the good to expand, not only in our consciousness, but also in the world. And there are many good things happening; for example, the tremendous growth in the vegan movement, greater social awareness of veganism, more plant-based products in the marketplace, and countless devoted advocates working to create a healthier and more compassionate world.

My survey respondents shared the power of hope. For example, one said, "I find encouragement and hope in witnessing how much my town has changed in adding vegan menu items and grocery store products, as well as inviting me to teach classes about veganism." Another explained, "I gain hope from the support from fellow vegans, activists, and advocates all working on the common goal of bringing about a world that actually works."

A practice that many find helpful for cultivating hope is to visualize a vegan world. Simply take a few minutes to picture what the world will look like and feel like if we all embrace the values of veganism and create a world of greater health, kindness, compassion, connection, and sustainability, a world where all have the potential to flourish.[18] Connect with your vision on a regular basis to bring hope and renewal. This helps to remind you of what you are working toward and what is possible. As noted by one survey respondent, "I feel better after visualizing the world I want to see. It helps me feel more peaceful, hopeful, and determined."

I close this chapter with the story of Rae Sikora, vegan for over forty-five years, author, activist, and humane educator.[19] Her story is a beautiful example of living her purpose, serving compassionately, and discovering the need to include herself in her circle of care. Her lived experience has led her to support other vegans with this same message.

Rae's story

Rae Sikora became vegetarian at age fifteen. She went to a leather shop with a friend and realized that leather was the skin of dead animals.

> I said out loud to my friend, "Don't buy anything in here. It's dead animals." I'd never met a vegetarian. I never knew there was such a thing. And then the woman behind the counter, who heard me, said, "Do you eat meat?" And then the light bulb went on. I had just eaten a hot dog. I turned to the woman at the counter. And I said, "No, I don't eat meat." After we left the shop, my friend asked, "Why did you lie to that woman?" And I said, "I didn't lie. I'll never eat meat again." That was the moment when I chose to align my values and my choices. And then it just grew from there.

She became vegan about five years later. She was renting space from a dairy farmer, and one day heard cows crying out loudly. When she went to see what was going on, new baby calves were being loaded onto a truck, with still-wet umbilical cords. The baby calves were crying for their mothers, and she could hear the mother cows in the barn calling out in distress. When she asked the owner of the farm what was going on, he explained that the male calves were being sent to a veal facility, because males were unnecessary for dairy production. She went to see the mother cows in the barn.

They were pressed up against the barbed wire, and just screaming, their mouths wide open. The barbed wire was cutting into them, and they were bleeding. It was horrible. When I came back out from behind the barn, I was crying. I said to the farmer, "I'm never going to consume dairy ever again." He said, "They get over it—and you'll get over it." But I said, "I don't want to get over it. I just witnessed something I shouldn't forget."

She began researching how her daily choices affected animals and the environment, which led her to stop consuming eggs. When she learned about the term *vegan* she said,

> I was so excited to learn there was a word for it, I wanted to scream it from the rooftops. Naively I thought it was a message people would be grateful to hear. Instead, people would say things like, "Don't be such a downer" when I told them about the harm caused by these industries. This didn't stop me, but it made me realize that adults were not necessarily interested in learning about this.

Rae started providing education in the schools, with the goal of teaching kids to cultivate critical thinking skills, question their assumptions about animals and nature, and learn new ways of relating to non-human animals. Initially, she did this on a volunteer basis, any time she had a day off from work. Eventually, she left her other jobs, and began doing this work full-time. She attended a Humane Education conference, where she was encouraged to present and share her work. This led to new opportunities and collaborations, and she later went on to co-create a certification training program in Humane Education with Zoe Weil, Ph.D.

Rae subsequently created workshops to help vegan activists and educators become more compassionate and effective communicators. She explained:

> I help activists communicate in ways that keep the heart door open, so that people are open to the message. I've realized, no one wants to join a community that makes them feel bad. People want to

feel welcome and invited. I teach activists, first of all, take care of yourself. We have to be an irresistible invitation to vegan living.

I worked with activists on what I call "despair repair." I began to examine what we are creating and co-creating together. When I looked at what causes despair, I realized that it's something that can be repaired. It's like the old Cherokee story of the two wolves who live inside of us. One works toward love, joy, and goodness and the other focuses on anger, resentment, and hatred. Which one will win? It's the wolf we are feeding.

I think we're each here to fulfill something. We're not just here to watch TV and go to the drive-thru and eat hamburgers; we're all here on our path. Some people are more consciously practicing a spiritual path. But I think everybody is on this path. I think our soul work is: "What am I doing between the time when I'm born and the time I die? And am I making the world a more loving place? Or am I adding to the suffering?" When I discovered this path of compassion, it gave me a purpose on this planet. Actually, I didn't discover it, it discovered me. I can spread love and compassion. I can't think of any other more worthwhile purpose.

Rae acknowledged that she has not always taken good care of herself. She learned to do this after discovering meditation and gaining more self-awareness. "I realized that if I'm physically healthy, making good choices for myself, it affects my mind, it affects my emotions, my movements, and my confidence in the world and who I am in the world. How can I be more effective in my outreach? I learned I need to be healthy and have good energy." She added:

I want to be aware, but sometimes it's painful. Sometimes despair catches me, at that point just between being awake and asleep. Sometimes I have flashback images of violence to animals that I witnessed. I have to make an effort to choose what brings me joy. I hike a lot. I spend a lot of time in the non-human world. I don't watch the news. I look at what is toxic for me and what nourishes me, and I keep a careful balance because I can go into despair way too easily.

I have learned that I don't have to always take in all the suffering, and that we are not really built for taking in as much as we do on social media and other outlets. We're in constant overload. I've realized that it's an ego thing if I think I can repair the world. I'm not the world's fixer. If I'm doing it to my own detriment, I'm not helping anyone. I used to feel I should work on activism all the time, and that doing the things I enjoyed was a luxury. I have learned that I need to do the things I love, like swimming and hiking. The more balanced I am, the more effective I am—so much more effective.

Lastly, Rae shared how vegan friendships have been an invaluable and uplifting part of her journey. "Being part of the vegan community has been really powerful for me. It's given me these deep meaningful relationships, a close community of people all over the world. It's great to have this sense of belonging to an amazing group of people who are thinking outside of themselves."

Hopefully, the tools, ideas, and experiences offered in this chapter have given you support, encouragement, and inspiration. If you wish to go deeper with any of the suggestions or practices, I invite you to check out the resources listed in this chapter and in the back of this book. The discovery that many of us make along our vegan journey is that the commitment to eating healthfully, compassionately, and sustainably has implications far beyond our own well-being. Join me in the next chapter to explore the larger impact of vegan living and how your personal healing journey helps to heal our world.

CHAPTER 11

MOVING TOWARD A COMPASSIONATE WORLD

"Nothing will benefit human health and the chance of survival
for life on Earth as much as the evolution to a vegetarian diet."
—**Albert Einstein**

"Your actions are so powerful, they'll touch people and animals
and forests and oceans you may never see."
—**Victoria Moran**, in *Main Street Vegan* [1]

The ripple effects of our healing

At its heart, veganism is about compassion. It's about making choices, through what we eat, what we purchase, and what we do, that lessen suffering for all sentient beings. As shown through the inspiring stories and examples throughout this book, a vegan lifestyle may ameliorate our own suffering as well—by reducing our risk for debilitating chronic disease, empowering us, and aligning us with our core values. It can strengthen our connection to ourselves and to other beings. We no longer need to close off our awareness to truths about the humane, ethical, health, and ecological costs of our animal-based food system. Veganism is a win–win solution that helps animals, wildlife, the environment, and our own physical and emotional well-being. It may well be the essential choice that heals our planet so that we and all beings can survive and thrive.

The choice to be vegan is, in and of itself, incredibly transformative. Mindfully choosing to eat plant-based, as an expression of care for animals, the environment, and our own well-being, brings a massive inner shift, along with saving the lives of sentient beings and living more lightly on the planet. The seven themes that were highlighted throughout this book can be transformative, whether you are vegan or not. Incorporating these principles and practices into your life can contribute to the holistic integration of mind, body, and spirit, and to a life that is more authentic, fulfilling, and impactful. When we bring these practices together—living or moving toward a vegan lifestyle, *alongside* our inner work to nurture mind, body, and spirit—the synergistic healing power can be exponential.

By integrating the *Seven Transformative Themes* into our vegan journey, we can flourish in mind, body, and spirit, and at the same time, send out positive ripples that create a healthier and more compassionate world. As I discuss in more depth next, the very principles that help us to heal and become our most authentic and fulfilled selves also bring more kindness, connection, and caring for others and the planet we all share.

Values alignment

As we take the time to clarify our core *values* and make daily choices that are in accord with these values, we feel truer to ourselves and more at peace. We discover the courage to listen to our inner knowing, to honor our conscience, and to course-correct when we discover that our actions are out of alignment or causing harm. We dare to be different, to be someone who leads by ethics of kindness, compassion, and generosity.

Cultivating compassion

As we broaden our *compassion*, we become willing to witness, care about, and, whenever possible, alleviate the suffering of others. We empathize with and try to understand others' feelings and perspectives, including those who seem different from us. We extend our compassion to all sentient beings, making choices that bring kindness, wholeness, and freedom for ourselves and others.

Deeper meaning and purpose

As we contribute our gifts toward causes that reflect our values, we experience genuine *meaning and purpose*. Our unique passions guide us to serve in ways that bring personal joy and positive impacts for others and our world. It doesn't matter whether we serve on a smaller scale in our family or local community, or on a larger, global scale—we each have a meaningful and essential purpose to fulfill.

Authentic fulfillment

As we learn to embrace the complexity of life and our emotional experience, we discover a more *authentic fulfillment*. We find that true well-being is not about "feeling good" all the time, but rather, embracing the diverse emotional milieu of life here on Planet Earth. We learn to care for ourselves through life's ups and downs, with holistic practices and meaningful activities that nourish our mind, body, and spirit. This grounded, authentic well-being helps us to live and give and serve from a space of flourishing rather than depletion.

True connection

As we build *meaningful connections*, we are encouraged and enriched by those who share our values, while at the same time learning the skills to peacefully navigate differences. Meaningful relationships help us to flourish, bring us joy, and strengthen us during times of discouragement. When we experience conflicts or differences, we learn to find common ground, communicate generatively, and build bridges of connection, rather than walls.

Health empowerment

As we take *charge of our health*, we find empowerment to live an active and vibrant life. Health is one of our most precious gifts, worth safeguarding through the best possible nutritional and lifestyle choices. Even though we all face the inevitability of aging and death, and the likelihood of some ailments along the way, empowerment is about taking action where we can. Our steps toward healthy living help others around us as well. Our vitality allows us to actively engage in life and relationships, and it inspires others to see what is possible.

Discovering our interconnectedness

And lastly, as we discover that we are all *interconnected*, with each other and with all of nature, we become more whole. We experience awe at the beauty and expansiveness of our world. We learn to listen to and trust our intuition, the inner voice that nudges and guides us. We sense that we are somehow connected with something or Someone larger than us, that holds this vastness and complexity. We realize that we are intricately connected with all beings, the universe, and galaxies beyond. We are connected in ways that we can't quite define and that bring a sense of wonder, mystery, and magic to our lives. Gradually, we see that caring for each part of this whole, intricate, interconnected system serves our own greatest well-being and the greatest good.

What's next?

In her book, *Radical Compassion*, psychologist and mindfulness teacher Tara Brach shares the wise words of a hospice worker, who summed up the greatest regret of the dying in this way: "I wish I'd had the courage to live a life true to myself." She invites us to reflect: "What does it mean to live true to yourself?"[2] What discoveries have *you* made about living truer to yourself, as you consider what you have taken from this book and your own reflections, insights, and actions along the way?

As you assimilate your discoveries from this journey, what are your next steps? What does *your* vegan transformation look like? What continued healing actions will help you to live most true to yourself? What does it look like and feel like to be the healthy, compassionate, loving, fulfilled, purposeful, and impactful person that you are and yearn to be? And as you continue your healing journey, what are the ripple effects for the larger world?

I invite you to revisit the visualization offered at the end of the last chapter: *Imagine a compassionate vegan world*. Envision what the world would be like if we all lived by values of compassion, peace, fairness, kindness, cooperation, collaboration, harmony, and justice. Perhaps if we truly lived by these values, together we could discover creative solutions that meet humanity's needs, while living in harmony with nature and all sentient beings. Through creative, innovative, and compassionate choices, we could heal the environment and climate, and nurture Mother Earth back to greater health and flourishing. Imagine, as part of this vision, being able to bring your truest self, contribute your gifts, and enjoy fulfilling and meaningful connections with other humans, animals, and our beautiful planet.

The idea of a compassionate, sustainable, and healthy world may seem highly aspirational, something to strive for, but very far off from our current reality. If you are like me, you may experience skepticism and cynicism—how could this type of global healing and peace ever happen? Yet healing and change often start through what we envision and allow ourselves to believe is possible. We hear and see enough negative messages and events in our world; while we must acknowledge and honor our feelings about these, we don't need to *cultivate* more negativity and hopelessness. When we examine what has contributed to positive social change in the past, it was often through the determination and hope-filled vision of a small number of leaders, who shared their vision and built positive momentum over time, gaining broader support and pioneering collaboration that created healing change.

With the immensity of need and suffering in our world, we may feel that there is little we can do to make a difference. We overlook the power of our presence and actions. Yet our choices and contributions often have an impact far beyond what we can see. As we have discussed throughout this book, making the choice to eat more compassionately and sustainably is a crucial contribution toward healing ourselves and our world. While we can't individually solve all the world's problems, we can choose, one meal at a time, to live in ways that increase kindness and justice while decreasing cruelty and suffering.

We have the power to live by our values, serve with our gifts, and share our voice to make a difference for what matters most to us. We can treat ourselves, one another, and all beings in ways that are aligned with the person we want to be, and the world we want to see. We can practice peaceful and heartful presence that has the power to open hearts and minds. Through our votes and advocacy, we can encourage lawmakers to move toward policies that are more just for all beings and the planet. We can become involved with organizations that share our passionate commitment and accomplish more through joining together than we ever could alone.

To create a healthier world, we must widen our circles of compassion. Vegan transformation involves caring for the well-being of all, extending kindness to all beings. And at the same time, our circle of compassion needs to include our own healing and well-being. When we witness the magnitude of unnecessary suffering in our world, it can be consuming and overwhelming. For those of us who are compassionate and empathic, those who are activists or advocates, and those who are caregivers or healers, it's especially important to include ourselves in our circle of care. We need to remember that our most lasting and meaningful impact comes from being the change we want to see—serving from a place of compassion and fullness, rather than burnout and depletion. We also need to remember our own limits and our own sphere of influence. I like to think of each of us as cells in the larger body, the larger whole, each with our own gifts, skills, and areas of contribution. We each have a part to play, but we can't do it all, and we can't do it alone.

As we hold these truths—that we can't do it all and yet we each play a crucial role in healing our world—we learn to balance contemplation and action, caring for self and caring for others, receiving and giving. In the process, we discover that these need not be separate or opposites— rather, in their healthiest forms, they all work together. As expressed by one research participant, "Through veganism, I feel that I'm making the best decisions for myself, for animals, and the future of our planet." You don't have to choose one or the other. As you transform yourself in the most aligned, aware, and compassionate ways, your presence and actions ripple out into expansive, all-encompassing tides of healing.

ACKNOWLEDGEMENTS

Researching and writing this book was a long, and at times intense, process—one influenced and inspired by many people who offered support and encouragement along the way. First, I want to thank all the amazing vegans who participated in my research surveys and interviews. Your actions, activism, words, and wisdom uplifted me and provided the foundation for many of the ideas shared in this book. I was moved by how your vegan journeys have impacted your own lives, and how you are each making this world a better place. Thank you for taking the time to complete my survey and share your experiences. For those of you whom I interviewed, thank you for meeting with me and telling your story, and for allowing it to be shared to inspire others.

I want to thank my many mentors, who have helped me believe in myself enough to bring my dream of writing a book into reality. First, much, much appreciation to Victoria Moran, my role model for being a vegan leader, who lives and embodies what she teaches. Thank you, Victoria, for Main Street Vegan Academy, which provided the foundational knowledge and the meaningful connections to start me on my own path as a vegan educator and contributor. I greatly appreciate your encouragement along the way, especially about writing this book.

Much appreciation to the following: Mitali Deypurkaystha (book mentor and founder of The Vegan Publisher)—your self-guided book writing course and your availability to answer questions were invaluable during the book planning, outlining, and initial phases of writing this book. Katrina Fox, for your vegan networking groups, your support, and connecting me with several people who participated in my research. Dr. Melanie Joy, for your encouragement about this book, and for being the vegan advocate, teacher, and leader that you are. You are a source of inspiration. Clare Mann (vegan psychologist and author), for offering your encouraging words and wise insights, and for your tireless vegan advocacy.

Dr. Claire Zammit, leader of Feminine Power and Women-Centered Coaching, whose training in transformational coaching and feminine leadership gave me the courage to honor my truth. I also appreciate the coaches who spurred me on to bring my vision for this book to fruition: Kate Ballo, Anna Kowalska, Lucie Malette, Stephanie Harter, and Sandra Nomoto.

I'm deeply grateful for friends who provided ongoing emotional support, insight, laughter, and wisdom through this whole process, including Rachael Leonard, Mariquita Solis, Marla Friedman, Sally Lipsky, Amie Hamlin, and Diana Goldman, along with many others. I appreciate my Feminine Power "sisters" from the Coaching and Leadership Programs who supported me throughout this endeavor. I'm also grateful to my parents and to my sisters, Cheryl and Teresa, for encouraging me to follow my dream to write. And I want to express appreciation to my stepdaughter, Lennay, for offering helpful research resources and encouragement.

Endless gratitude and appreciation go to my husband, Dennis Chapman. Without your emotional and practical support, I'm not sure this book could have happened. Thank you for listening and being a loving support on my journey, and for going on the journey with me. Thank you for bringing your expertise as a social work educator to review and offer editing suggestions for each and every chapter. Your feedback and insights were invaluable. There are no words to express my appreciation and how much you mean to me.

Lastly, I am so appreciative to be working with Lantern Publishing & Media. Lantern has published the books of many leaders and teachers I greatly admire, and I'm honored to now be included in the Lantern family. Thank you to Brian Normoyle and the Lantern team for believing in me and the book's message, and helping to make this book a reality.

A final word: For my readers, thank you for diving into this book and taking what resonates into your own life and out into the world.

RECIPES AND MEAL IDEAS

What does one eat on a vegan diet? I used to wonder that, too. Since going plant-based, I have come to realize the abundance of delicious plant-based options. What has been most astonishing for me (and for many vegans) is the discovery that my food options expanded greatly—and became more varied, delectable, *and* healthy—when I moved to a plant-exclusive diet.

In this section, I will share some vegan recipes contributed by my research participants. But first, let's talk about a few everyday options that don't necessarily require a recipe. I list some common meal ideas that can easily be "veganized." For lunch and dinner options, consider adding beans, lentils, tofu, tempeh, or mushrooms (in place of meat or fish). Explore varieties of plant-based milk, cheese, and yogurt to substitute for cow's milk products. Include a colorful array of veggies, fruits, and leafy greens as often as possible. And then add your favorite (vegan) seasonings, spices, sauces, and condiments for flavor.

Breakfast Ideas

- Oatmeal, fruit, and nuts
- Muesli (rolled oats soaked in plant-based milk) with fruit, dates, and nuts
- Granola with plant-based milk and fruit
- Plant-based yogurt and fruit
- Whole grain bread or sprouted grain bread with peanut butter or almond butter
- Avocado toast (toast with vegan mayonnaise and avocado slices)
- Cashew French toast (soak 3 pieces of bread in a blended mixture of 1/4 cup ground cashews, 1/2 teaspoon cinnamon, and 1/2 cup plant-based milk, then cook the soaked bread in a non-stick pan over medium heat until browned on both sides. Serve with fruit and maple syrup).

- Smoothie (blended with fruit, plant-based milk or water, a handful of greens, and other ingredients and flavorings as desired. Also see smoothie recipes included later).

Lunch and Dinner Ideas

- Large salad with greens, veggies, fruit, beans, nuts, and/or seeds
- Stir-fried or sauteed veggies over quinoa, couscous, brown rice, or other whole grain
- Soup (lentil, veggie, curry, black bean, minestrone—the options are endless)
- Wrap with hummus and veggies
- Power bowl with veggies, quinoa or rice, legumes, and dressing or sauce
- Pasta with marinara, pesto, or other sauce
- Falafel on pita or on salad with tahini dressing
- Hummus or baba ganoush (eggplant spread) on pita and/or with veggies
- Veggie and bean burritos, tacos, quesadillas, or enchiladas
- Veggie pizza (with extra sauce and veggies, using no cheese or plant-based cheese)
- Veggie burgers, bean burgers, or marinated portobello mushrooms on the stove or grill
- Grilled sandwich with veggies, guacamole, and/or plant-based cheese
- Veggie lasagna (use plant-based cheese or tofu "ricotta" instead of dairy cheese)

Plant-Powered Recipes

Here are recipes from my amazing vegan culinary contributors. Some of the recipes are free of salt, oil, and/or sugar, while others are not. Depending on your tastes, health needs, etc., feel free to adjust the recipes with your favorite seasonings to create the flavors you like. Over time, you may find that you need less salt, sugar, or oil to create delicious-tasting food. For more vegan recipes, check out the cookbooks listed in the Resources section of this book. In addition, many of the websites shared in the Resources have great (free) recipes you can enjoy.

Breakfast Recipes

Tofu Scramble with Mushroom & Basil

From Diana Goldman

This protein-rich, cholesterol-free scramble is my go-to for overnight guests—both friends and family. It's dressed up with umami-packed mushrooms, slightly sweet and earthy kale, and a variety of spices. A sprinkling of fresh basil elevates the flavor to the next level.—Diana

Ingredients

- 14-ounce package firm or extra-firm tofu, drained
- 2 Tbsp nutritional yeast
- 1 tsp sea salt
- 1/2 tsp ground black pepper
- 1/2 tsp ground cumin
- 1/2 tsp ground turmeric
- 2 cups destemmed chopped kale
- 3/4 cup halved cherry tomatoes
- 1 Tbsp olive oil
- 1 small yellow onion, diced
- 3 cloves garlic, minced
- 8 ounces white, baby bella, button, cremini, or portobello mushrooms, sliced
- 1/4 cup fresh basil, sliced into chiffonade (thin ribbons)
- Hot sauce, freshly squeezed lemon juice, diced avocado, salsa, and/or nutritional yeast (optional, for serving)

Directions

1. In a medium mixing bowl, crumble the tofu until no large pieces remain. Add the nutritional yeast, salt, pepper, cumin, and turmeric and stir until well combined. Add the kale and tomatoes.
2. Heat the oil in a large skillet over medium-high heat. Add the onions and a pinch of salt. Cook for 4–6 minutes or until softened. Add the garlic and sauté for 30 seconds. Add the mushrooms and cook for 6

minutes, or until their moisture releases and cooks off and they begin to soften and brown.

3. Add the crumbled tofu mixture to the skillet and cook for 5–6 minutes, stirring occasionally, or until the tofu is heated through and the kale has wilted. If the mixture starts to stick while cooking, turn down the heat or add a splash of water. Turn off the heat and stir in the basil.
4. Serve hot with optional toppings, if desired.

Crunchy Granola
From Angela Crawford

Ingredients

- 2 cups rolled oats (uncooked)
- 1 1/2 to 2 cups nuts (I use a combination of almonds, cashews, pecans, and walnuts, about 1/2 cup each)
- 3 Tbsp pumpkin seeds (and/or sunflower or sesame seeds)
- 1/2 cup shredded coconut
- 1 1/2 tsp cinnamon
- 1 Tbsp cacao powder (optional)
- 1 Tbsp ground flax seed (optional)
- 1/3 cup maple syrup
- 2 Tbsp almond butter (optional)
- 1/2 cup raisins or chopped dates (optional)

Directions

1. Preheat the oven to 375 °F. If using almond butter, stir it into 1/3 cup maple syrup; blend until creamy.
2. Mix all ingredients in a large bowl, except for the raisins or dates, and spread on a large, rimmed baking sheet lined with parchment paper.
3. Bake for about 15 minutes (check after 10 minutes and adjust timing depending on desired level of crunchiness. I like crunchy granola, so sometimes I bake it for 20 minutes.)

4. Add 1/2 cup raisins or chopped dates (if desired) to the warm granola. Let granola rest on the baking sheet for about 15 minutes to cool. It will get crunchier as it cools.
5. Serve with plant-based milk or yogurt, and fruit.

Apple Walnut Quinoa Breakfast Bowl
From Pascale Dantes

Ingredients

- 1 cup quinoa, rinsed and drained
- 2 cups water
- 1 diced (or grated) apple
- 1 tsp cinnamon
- 2 to 4 Tbsp walnut halves (optional)
- 1 tsp raw cacao nibs (optional)
- 1 Tbsp raisins, chopped dates, or dried cranberries (optional)

Directions

1. In a saucepan, add the quinoa, water, apple, and cinnamon. Bring to a boil over medium-high heat.
2. Reduce heat to low, cover, and simmer for 15 minutes or until the quinoa is cooked. Remove from heat and stir in the walnuts.
3. Serve warm, and top with raw cacao nibs and raisins, if desired.
4. Note: For a creamier quinoa, substitute plant-based milk for some of the water or add plant-based milk to the cooked quinoa. If you don't like the chunkiness of the quinoa, place the cooked quinoa in a food processor with 1/4 to 1/2 cup plant-based milk and blend to desired consistency before adding optional toppings.

Go-To Green Smoothie
From Karen Ranzi

Ingredients

- 1 large apple, chopped
- 1 large mango or frozen mango, chopped
- 1 cup or more wild blueberries
- Leafy green of choice (I use about 8 leaves of kale)
- 1 1/2 cups water (adjust depending on desired consistency)

Directions

1. Blend all ingredients until smooth.

50+ Muscle Booster Smoothie Bowl
From Karin Wentworth-Ping

Ingredients

- 1/2 cup (100ml) plant-based milk
- 2 very ripe bananas
- 1 mango
- 2 Tbsp plant-based yogurt and/or silken tofu
- Handful of blackberries (or other berries or chopped fruit)
- 1 Tbsp mixed seeds (e.g., sunflower, pumpkin, chia, sesame, and/or ground flaxseed)
- Dried cranberries (optional)
- Shredded coconut (optional)
- Sprinkle of magnesium (optional)

Directions

1. Put the bananas, mango, plant milk, yogurt or tofu, and magnesium (optional) into a blender (or use an immersion blender). Don't blend the berries in with the other ingredients, otherwise the smoothie will be gray. Blend until creamy.

2. Play with the amount of plant-based milk and yogurt/tofu to make it thicker or thinner, adjusting it to your liking.

3. Add the blackberries (or any berries or fruit), seed mix, dried cranberries, and coconut on top.

No Oatmeal Cereal
From Karen Ranzi

Ingredients

- 2 to 3 bananas, chopped
- 2 to 3 apples, chopped
- 2 medjool dates (soaked if not soft), chopped
- 1 tsp or more cinnamon
- 3 Tbsp raisins, soaked 2 hours
- Optional: Handful of blueberries or other fruit

Directions

1. Process bananas, apples, dates, and cinnamon in a food processor or blender until the mixture reaches an oatmeal-like consistency. Add soaked raisins and any optional ingredients, then stir.

Chickpea Flour Omelet with Vegetables
From Pascale Dantes

Ingredients

- 1 cup chickpea (garbanzo bean) flour
- 2 Tbsp nutritional yeast flakes
- 1/2 tsp turmeric powder
- 1/2 tsp garlic powder
- 1/2 tsp baking powder
- 1/4 to 1/2 tsp salt
- Pinch of ground black pepper
- 1 cup water

- 1 tsp apple cider vinegar
- 1 cup chopped mushrooms
- 1 red bell pepper, diced
- 1/2 cup chopped spring onion (bulb and stalk)

Directions

1. In a medium bowl, combine the dry ingredients: chickpea flour, nutritional yeast flakes, turmeric, garlic powder, baking powder, salt, and pepper. Once the dry ingredients are mixed, stir in water and apple cider vinegar. Mix until smooth and a pancake-like batter has formed, then set aside. Let rest for 10 to 15 minutes while cooking the vegetables.
2. Heat a nonstick pan over medium heat and coat with a small amount of spray oil. Cook the mushrooms and red peppers in the pan until softened. Remove from the pan and set aside.
3. Wipe the pan clean and spray again lightly with oil. Pour in the chickpea flour batter and spread it out to form a large "pancake." (If the batter is too thick to spread easily, add 1 to 2 Tbsp water and stir).
4. Place a lid over the pan and cook the omelet over medium heat for 3 minutes or until lightly browned. Flip the omelet and cook for 2 more minutes.
5. Once cooked, place the omelet on a plate and fill it with mushrooms and peppers, and fold. Sprinkle with chopped spring onion.

Note: Feel free to add any other sautéed or raw vegetables as desired (e.g., zucchini, spinach, tomatoes). Delicious topped with salsa, guacamole, or vegan cream cheese as well.

Lunch and Dinner Recipes

Marinated Tempeh & Sweet Potato Wrap

From Diana Goldman

Ingredients

- 1 medium sweet potato, cooked
- 8-ounce package tempeh
- 1/4 cup soy sauce or tamari
- 2 Tbsp maple syrup
- 2 cloves garlic, minced
- 1 1/2 tsp dried rosemary
- 1 tsp ground black pepper
- 4 whole wheat wraps (about 12-inch in size)
- 1/2 cup hummus
- 2 cups destemmed chopped kale, loosely packed

Directions

1. Place the tempeh flat on a cutting board and slice into thin strips.
2. In an 8 x 8-inch glass baking dish or other flat-bottomed dish, stir to combine the soy sauce or tamari, maple syrup, garlic, rosemary, and pepper. Add the tempeh and flip it over a few times to coat.
3. Heat a medium skillet over medium-high heat. Add the tempeh with the marinade and cook for 3–4 minutes, or until all the marinade has evaporated and the tempeh is a deep golden color with a sticky coating. Don't leave the skillet unwatched, as this is a fast process.
4. Place one wrap on a cutting board. Spread with 2 tablespoons of hummus, 2 tablespoons of sweet potato, 4 slices of tempeh, and 1/2 cup of kale. Fold in the sides, fold up the bottom, then roll upwards to close the wrap. Slice into halves. Repeat with the remaining wraps.

Eggplant Patties with Tahini Dressing

From Wanda Huberman, National Health Association (NHA)

Tahini Dressing

Ingredients

- Juice of 3 to 4 oranges, lemons, and/or limes
- 1/2 cup of tahini
- Handful of cashews
- 1 peeled shallot

Directions

1. Blend all ingredients in a blender or food processor until creamy. Add more cashews, juice, or tahini for desired thickness or flavor. If the dressing is too thick, you can thin it with 1 to 2 Tbsp water. This sauce can be used as a salad dressing or topping.

Eggplant Patties

Ingredients

- 2 large eggplants, peeled and cubed
- 3 stalks of celery, chopped
- 1 large yellow or white onion, peeled and chopped
- 1/2 cup cashews and 1/2 cup almonds

Directions

1. Steam the eggplants, celery, and onion until soft (about 10 to 15 minutes). Place steamed vegetables in a bowl and chop them into small pieces, creating a batter. Alternatively, you can pulse the vegetables briefly in the food processor.
2. Grind cashews and almonds in a blender or food processor. Stir the ground nuts into the vegetable batter. Place the batter in a covered bowl and refrigerate overnight.
3. Form into patties. (If they don't hold together well, mix additional ground cashews or almond flour into the batter).

4. Bake on parchment paper for 15–20 minutes at 375 °F or until firm and brown enough to turn over with a spatula; bake the other side. Bake about 15 to 20 minutes per side.

5. Drizzle patties with tahini dressing and serve.

The Whole Enchilada

From Amie Hamlin, Coalition for Healthy School Food (CHSF)

(Recipe developed by Chef David Stroka, Chef Manager, Binghamton, NY City School District, for CHSF)

Ingredients

- 1 Tbsp water, or more as needed (or 1 tsp olive oil)
- 1 cup chopped onions
- 1 or 2 garlic cloves, pressed or minced
- 1/2 green or red bell pepper, stemmed, seeded, and diced
- 1 Tbsp ground cumin
- 2 cups peeled, shredded sweet potato or winter squash (Note: 2 small to medium sweet potatoes or 1 1/2 pound butternut squash should yield about 2 cups shredded)
- 3 cups cooked kidney or pinto beans (two 15-oz cans, drained)
- 28-oz can of enchilada sauce or tomato sauce
- Salt and pepper, to taste (optional)
- 12 whole wheat tortillas (8-inch size)

Directions

1. Preheat the oven to 375 °F. Lightly oil two 8 x 8-inch or 9 x 9-inch pans.

2. For the filling, in a large saucepan on medium heat, cook the onions in water or oil until soft, about 4 minutes. Stir in the garlic, bell peppers, and cumin, and cook for 3 or 4 minutes, until the peppers soften. Add the shredded sweet potatoes or squash and cook, stirring frequently, for about 5 minutes, until hot. Add the beans and stir well.

3. Cover the bottoms of the baking pans with enchilada or tomato sauce about 1/4-inch deep. Working on a dry surface, place a

generous 1/2 cup of filling a little off center on the first tortilla. Lift the shorter edge up and over the filling and roll up the tortilla with just enough pressure to spread the filling close to the ends (without pushing any out). Place the enchilada up against one side of the baking pan. Continue rolling enchiladas and filling the pans, six to a pan. They should fit snugly. Spread the rest of the sauce evenly over the enchiladas.

4. Cover the pans with foil and bake for about 30 minutes, until thoroughly hot. To serve, use a spatula to lift enchiladas out of the pan and onto dinner plates.

Summer Couscous Salad
From Pascale Dantes

Ingredients

- 1 cup couscous
- 1 1/2 cup water (or amount recommended on couscous package instructions)
- 1 orange bell pepper
- 3 cucumbers
- 1 Tbsp apple cider vinegar
- Juice of 1 lime
- 1/4 to 1/2 tsp salt (to taste)

Directions

1. Prepare couscous according to package instructions. Fluff cooked couscous with a fork.
2. Meanwhile, dice the bell pepper and cucumber into small cubes. In a separate bowl, whisk together the apple cider vinegar, lime juice, and salt.
3. Once the couscous has cooled, add the diced vegetables and dressing. Stir to combine and serve chilled. Adjust seasonings as desired.

Note: Add other raw vegetables as desired, such as shredded red cabbage, shredded carrot, or chopped celery.

Quinoa Stuffed Bell Peppers

From Pascale Dantes

Ingredients

- 2 or 3 red bell peppers
- 1 cup cooked quinoa
- 1 small onion, diced
- 1 tsp taco seasoning
- 1 1/2 cup organic black beans
- 1 cup tomatoes, diced
- 1 celery stalk, diced
- 1 Tbsp olive oil

Directions

1. Preheat the oven to 375 °F. Cut the bell peppers in half and remove the seeds.
2. In a bowl, combine the cooked quinoa, onions, seasoning mix, black beans, tomatoes, and celery. Add olive oil and mix until everything is combined.
3. Spoon the quinoa mixture into the bell pepper halves. Place the peppers in a baking dish and cover with aluminum foil. Bake for 25 minutes. Remove the foil and bake for an additional 5 minutes.
4. Serve and enjoy.

Not Tuna Salad

From Karen Ranzi

Ingredients

- 1 cup walnuts or sunflower seeds, soaked a few hours, drained, and rinsed
- 1/2 cup celery, chopped
- 1/2 cup red pepper, chopped
- 1/4 cup parsley, chopped
- 2 tsp minced onion
- Juice from 1/2 lime
- 1/2 Tbsp dulse flakes (to taste)

Directions

1. Process all ingredients in your food processor until you reach a chunky, but well-combined texture.
2. Serve on a large bed of lettuce or stuffed in tomatoes or bell peppers, along with a large main meal green salad.

Cauliflower Tabouleh

From Karen Ranzi

Ingredients

- 1/2 large cauliflower, chopped (or one whole small cauliflower)
- One large bunch parsley, chopped
- One large tomato, diced
- 3 scallions, diced
- 1/2 cup lemon juice
- Several sprigs of mint if available
- One avocado, diced
- One cucumber, diced (optional)
- Salt and pepper (to taste, optional)

Directions

1. Process cauliflower in the food processor with an S blade until well ground. Remove the cauliflower from the food processor and place in a large bowl.
2. Process parsley, tomato, scallions, lemon juice and mint. Pulse several times until well mixed. Stir together with cauliflower.
3. Add diced avocado and/or cucumber and stir thoroughly.

Basil Lime Pesto on Raw Zucchini Noodles
From Karen Ranzi

Ingredients

- 2 large zucchini, made into zucchini noodles with a spiralizer or pasta hand tool
- 3 cups fresh basil, stems removed
- 1 bunch parsley
- 1/2 cup walnuts (or mixture of walnuts and pine nuts)
- 1/2 cup water
- 1/2 tsp dulse flakes
- 1/4 cup fresh-squeezed lime juice

Directions

1. Place zucchini noodles on a plate.
2. To make basil lime pesto, combine all other ingredients in a food processor or blender until desired consistency is achieved. You may need to add more or less dulse depending on taste.
3. Serve basil lime pesto on zucchini noodles.

Note: If you prefer cooked, rather than raw, zucchini noodles, lightly heat them in a pan to desired tenderness.

Spicy Carrot Ginger Soup
From Angela Crawford

Ingredients

- 2 to 3 cups of chopped carrots (about 6 medium carrots)
- 1 large onion (diced)
- 4 cups water
- 1/2 cup raw cashews, soaked for 2 hours, drained, and rinsed
- 2 to 3 tsp curry powder (to taste)
- 1 to 2 tsp fresh grated ginger

- 2 Tbsp soy sauce or Braggs Liquid Aminos
- Salt and pepper, as needed
- Cilantro for garnish (or parsley)

Directions

1. In a large soup pot, combine the carrots, onions, and water. Add the curry powder and ginger. Cover and bring to a boil, then turn down the heat and simmer for 10–15 minutes until vegetables are tender.
2. Place the cooked vegetables, cooking liquid, cashews, and soy sauce into the blender and blend until creamy. You may have to do this in batches, depending on the size of your blender. If the soup is too thick, add more water. Adjust seasonings as desired. (Add optional salt and pepper as desired).
3. Serve hot and garnish with parsley or cilantro.

Pumpkin and Black Bean Soup

From Angela Crawford

Ingredients

- 1 medium onion, peeled and finely diced
- 4 cups water or vegetable broth
- 1 can (14 ounces) diced tomatoes in juice
- 1 can (15 ounces) pumpkin puree
- 1/2 cup red lentils, rinsed
- 1 can (15 ounces) black beans, drained and rinsed
- 2 tsp curry powder
- 1 tsp ground cumin
- 1/4 tsp cayenne (optional – add last if desire more "heat")
- 1 tsp salt (to taste)
- 1/2 cup plant-based milk (e.g., soy or almond milk)

Directions

1. Sauté onion in 1 Tbsp of olive oil or water for about 10 minutes over medium heat, until tender. Add the curry and cumin and sauté for about 30 seconds.
2. Add broth, pumpkin, diced tomatoes, and red lentils. Turn up the heat and bring to a boil. Then cover the pot, reduce the heat to medium, and cook for 20–25 minutes, until the lentils are tender.
3. Puree 2–3 cups of the soup in the blender, then return to the pot. Add the black beans and plant-based milk, along with salt and optional cayenne pepper to taste. If the soup is too thick, add a little water as needed. Simmer for 5 minutes, adjust seasonings, and serve.

White Bean Chili

From Angela Crawford

Ingredients

- 1 onion, peeled and diced
- 1 bell pepper, seeded and diced (red, orange, or green, depending on preference)
- 1 carrot, grated or chopped
- 3 cloves garlic, peeled and minced
- 2 tsp ground cumin
- 1 tsp chili powder
- 1 tsp oregano
- 1/4 tsp cayenne (optional)
- 28-oz can diced tomatoes
- 4 cups (or two 15-oz cans) cooked white beans, drained and rinsed
- 3 cups vegetable stock or water
- Juice of 1 lime
- Finely chopped cilantro (about 1/2 cup)
- 1 tsp salt (or adjust to taste)
- Avocado slices (optional)

Directions

1. Place the onion, pepper, and carrot in a large saucepan and sauté over medium heat for about 10 minutes, until soft. Add water 1 to 2 Tbsp at a time to keep from sticking to the pan. Add garlic and spices (cumin, chili powder, oregano, and optional cayenne) and cook for 30 seconds, stirring frequently.
2. Add the tomatoes, beans, and vegetable stock (or water). Bring to a boil over high heat. Reduce the heat to medium and cook, covered, for 20–30 minutes.
3. If you prefer a creamier soup, puree about 2 cups of the soup in the blender, then return to the pot and stir. Add the lime juice and salt. Adjust seasonings as desired.
4. Garnish with cilantro and optional avocado slices, then serve.

Beet Burgers
From Angela Crawford

Ingredients

- 2 raw medium sized beets
- 1 cup rolled oats
- 2 cups (one 15-oz can) beans (aduki or pinto beans work well)
- 2 cloves minced garlic
- 1 flax "egg" (Mix 1 Tbsp flax meal with 3 Tbsp water and allow to sit for 5 minutes, until it reaches a gel-like consistency.)
- Spices as desired (I use a dash of spices such as parsley, thyme, basil, chili powder, and/or smoked paprika, 1 to 2 tsp total)
- Salt and pepper to taste

Directions

1. Process the oats in a food processor until ground into flour. Set aside.
2. Peel the raw beets and shred or grate them in the food processor. Add 1/2 cup of the oat flour and the remaining ingredients (beans, flax "egg," garlic, spices, salt, and pepper). Pulse until combined, then stir in the remaining flour.

3. Form into patties. If you have time, it can be helpful to refrigerate the batter for a few hours (to help the patties hold together better).

4. Heat a pan with a teaspoon of olive oil and cook over medium heat for about 3 minutes per side. (Alternatively, bake the patties on a baking sheet for 10 to 15 minutes per side at 375 °F).

Note: I often freeze any extra burgers, and then grill or re-heat them on a skillet or grill when ready for use. The beet burgers always get rave reviews at cookouts!

Awesome Bean Burgers

From Amie Hamlin, Coalition for Healthy School Food (CHSF)
(Recipe developed by Chef Wynnie Stein of Moosewood Restaurant for CHSF)

Ingredients

- 3 cups cooked black beans, drained (two 15-oz cans or 1 1/2 cups dried)
- 1 medium sweet potato, steamed or baked until soft
- 1 Tbsp tomato paste
- 1/2 cup quick-cooking oats (or rolled oats briefly whirled in a blender)
- 2 tsp soy sauce
- 1 tsp ground cumin
- 1 tsp chili powder
- 1 tsp garlic powder
- 1 tsp Dijon-style mustard
- 1/4 tsp salt
- 1/4 tsp ground black pepper

Directions

1. Preheat oven to 350 °F. Line a baking sheet with parchment paper or lightly oil it.

2. In a food processor, pulse the black beans, cooked sweet potato (remove the skin), tomato paste, and oats until well combined. Mix the remaining ingredients in a small bowl, then add to the food processor and pulse again until combined. Alternatively, mash the

beans with a potato masher or large fork, then mash in the sweet potato and oats. Add the rest of the ingredients and stir well.

3. Form the mixture into 6 patties. Place the patties on the prepared baking sheet and bake until brown on one side, 8–10 minutes. Flip and bake for 10 more minutes.

4. Serve while hot, in a bun or not. Add your favorite toppings. Leftovers make a great snack served cold or reheated.

Celery Leaf Pesto
From Karin Wentworth-Ping

Ingredients

- 2 cups celery leaves
- 1/4 cup pumpkin and sunflower seeds
- 1/4 cup walnuts
- 1/4 cup extra virgin olive oil
- 1/4 to 1/2 cup nutritional yeast flakes
- 1/4 cup fresh lemon juice
- Water, optional if needed
- Salt and pepper, to taste

Directions

1. In a blender, first blend the celery leaves into a paste.

2. Scrape paste from the sides of the blender, then add all the other ingredients. Blend on high. You might need to scrape the sides occasionally to get a good even mix. Adjust to your preferred taste and texture by adding or decreasing the amount of garlic, lemon juice, and yeast flakes.

3. If using this recipe for a pasta dish, add some water gradually when blending, until it's smooth but not runny. Not keen on using oil? Add more nuts and seeds instead.

Note: Celery leaves are usually discarded but have a variety of nutrients as well as fiber and make a delicious addition to this pesto. This recipe can also be used as a dip or spread. If you do not have enough celery leaves, you can add or substitute basil or parsley leaves.

Desserts and Snacks

Vegan Vanilla Cupcakes

From Karin Wentworth-Ping

Cupcake Ingredients

- 1 3/4 cups all-purpose flour
- 1 cup white granulated sugar
- 1 tsp baking soda
- 1/4 tsp salt
- 1 cup soy or other plant milk
- 1/3 cup vegetable oil
- 2 tsp vanilla extract
- 1 Tbsp distilled white vinegar

Icing Ingredients

- 1/2 cup vegan butter, slightly softened
- 3 cups icing sugar (powdered sugar)
- 2 tsp vanilla extract
- Sprinkles, optional

Cupcake Directions

1. Preheat the oven to 350 °F. Line a 12-cup muffin pan with paper or silicone liners.
2. Sift the flour into a bowl and add the sugar, baking soda, and salt. Mix well.
3. Add the soy milk, vanilla extract, oil, and white vinegar. Whisk by hand (or use an electric mixer on low) to a smooth, runny consistency.
4. Pour or scoop the batter evenly into the cupcake liners. Bake for 20–25 minutes until golden on top. Check the cupcakes at 20 minutes. Insert a toothpick into the center. If it doesn't come out clean, bake for 5 more minutes.
5. Move to a cooling rack and allow cupcakes to cool thoroughly before frosting.

Icing Directions

1. In a large mixing bowl, blend the vegan butter and vanilla with an electric mixer until smooth. Gradually add the icing sugar, 1/2 cup at a time, and start mixing at low, then increase to medium, until all blended in with a smooth texture.
2. Pipe or spoon onto the cooled cupcakes. Decorate with sprinkles or fresh strawberries, then serve.

Peanut Butter/Dried Cherry/Chocolate Chip Cookies

From Wanda Huberman, NHA

Ingredients

- 1 1/2 cup old-fashioned oats
- 12 Medjool dates—pitted and chopped (if dates are hard, soak for a couple of hours in warm water for easier blending)
- 1/2 cup roasted peanut butter
- 1/2 cup shredded unsweetened coconut (or coconut flakes)
- 1/2 cup unsweetened applesauce (you can substitute a very ripe banana)
- 1 Tbsp of cacao powder
- 1 Tbsp vanilla extract
- 1 Tbsp apple cider vinegar
- 1 tsp baking soda
- 1/2 cup dried unsulfured and unsweetened dark sweet cherries (can substitute raisins)
- 1/2 cup dairy-free dark chocolate chips (if unavailable, chop a 100% baking bar).

Directions

1. Preheat the oven to 350 °F. In a small bowl, mix the baking soda, apple cider vinegar, and vanilla extract and set aside.
2. In a food processor or blender, pulse oats until a fine flour forms.
3. Combine the oat flour, shredded coconut, cacao powder, peanut butter, dates, apple sauce, and baking soda mixture in the food processor and

pulse until a concentrated, sticky dough forms. (Alternatively, you can blend the wet ingredients and dates in the food processor, then mix in the flour, shredded coconut, and cacao by hand.)

4. Place the preceding contents in a large mixing bowl, add the 1/2 cup of chocolate chips and dried cherries, and mix by hand. (This must be done by hand because the dough will be too thick to mix with a spoon. Optionally, you may chop the chocolate chips and dried cherries)

5. Scoop twelve 2–3 tablespoon-size pieces of dough and mold into round disk-shaped cookies and place them on a cookie sheet lined with parchment paper.

6. Bake for 12–15 minutes. Let cool at least 10 minutes prior to eating.

7. They can be stored for at least a week out of refrigeration in a sealed glass container. They also keep very well in the freezer.

Oatmeal-Raisin Almond Butter alternative: Follow the same process, substituting roasted almond butter for peanut butter in the dough mixture, then a half cup of raisins and a half cup of old-fashioned oats in place of the chocolate chips and dried cherries.

Chocolate Cherry Smoothie
From Wanda Huberman, NHA

Ingredients

- 2 cups water (or more as needed)
- 2–3 cups of kale, spinach, or other leafy greens (or more as desired)
- 2–3 tsp seeds (e.g., mixture of ground flax, chia, and/or hemp seeds)
- 2 cups frozen cherries
- 1/2 to 1 frozen banana
- 1–2 Tbsp cacao powder
- 1 chopped date (optional)

Directions

1. Place 2 cups of water into a blender (add more or less, depending on desired thickness).

2. Fill the remainder of the blender with greens.

3. *If you are new to adding greens to your smoothie, start with 2–3 cups and add more to taste.
4. Add ground seeds (e.g., flax, chia, and hemp).
5. Blend ingredients to provide more room in the blender.
6. Add frozen cherries, frozen banana, cacao powder, and optional chopped date.
7. Blend until smooth.

Almond Chocolate Bars
From Angela Crawford

Ingredients

- 1/3 cup rolled oats
- 1/2 cup raw almonds
- 1/4 cup pumpkin seeds
- 2 Tbsp sesame or sunflower seeds
- 2 Tbsp ground flax seeds
- 1 Tbsp chia seeds
- 1 Tbsp hemp seeds
- 1/4 cup unsweetened coconut flakes
- 1/3 cup chocolate chips (dairy-free)
- 1/3 cup almond butter
- 1/4 cup agave syrup

Directions

1. Heat the oven to 350 °F. Spread oats, almonds, pumpkin seeds, and sesame or sunflower seeds on a baking sheet. Toast until golden, stirring occasionally, for about 7–10 minutes.
2. Cool, then place in a large bowl. Stir in the chocolate chips, coconut, flax meal, chia, and hemp seeds. In a small bowl, stir together the almond butter and agave syrup, then add to the other ingredients and mix well.
3. Spread in a 9 x 9 baking dish lined with parchment paper. Cover tightly and refrigerate for an hour or longer to firm up.
4. Cut into bars and keep refrigerated until served.

Recipe Contributors

Pascale Dantes

Pascale is a certified vegan health and life coach, meditation coach, and culinary expert who guides her clients to create mouthwatering, healthy, plant-based meals. Pascale adopted a plant-based, vegan lifestyle to help manage autoimmune disease. Before becoming vegan, she had frequent flare-ups. Through her vegan lifestyle, she found a powerful tool that has reduced symptoms and dramatically improved her quality of life. Now, she coaches and guides others in their transition to a vegan lifestyle. Pascale authored the cookbook *My Vegan Flow*. To learn more about Pascale's work, go to www.myveganflow.com.

Diana Goldman

Diana is the author of the *Plants For You Cookbook*. She is a chef, food photographer, and plant-based nutrition educator based in Boston, Massachusetts. She is the creator of BeantownKitchen.com, named one of the top 100 plant-based blogs by Feedspot. She has presented on plant-based eating for numerous companies, organizations, and institutions, and has been awarded grants from Harvard Pilgrim Healthcare to teach healthy cooking classes in the Boston area. Her recipes and articles have been featured in *VEGWORLD Magazine*, *Forks Over Knives*, and *Nourish Magazine*. Diana earned a B.S. in nutritional sciences from Cornell University and a master's degree in education from Harvard University. She adopted a plant-based lifestyle in 2013. Learn more about Diana at www.BeantownKitchen.com.

Amie Hamlin

Amie is co-founder and executive director of the Coalition for Healthy School Food (CHSF). CHSF is a nonprofit that promotes plant-based foods and nutrition education in schools to teach the whole community about the effects of our food choices on health, the environment, equity, and other social justice issues. Learn more about CHSF at www.

healthyschoolfood.org. Amie is also the founder of ClubVeg, a local veg group located in the Ithaca and Binghamton, New York area, that has offered educational programs, restaurant outings, and plant-based Grand Rounds for doctors at hospitals, and currently focuses on veganic agriculture. Amie raised her now adult daughter as a vegan since birth. She is passionate about the benefits of a plant-powered, vegan lifestyle and has been vegan since 1989.

Wanda Huberman

Wanda is the executive director of the National Health Association (NHA). She retired from her previous work of thirty years in the casualty insurance industry to work full-time with the NHA alongside her husband, Mark Huberman (president of NHA). The NHA is the longest-running nonprofit vegan organization in the United States. Founded in 1948, the NHA promotes the benefits of a whole-food, plant-exclusive diet. It provides an annual conference (with inspiring presenters and delicious plant-based meals), educational magazine, biweekly newsletter, and weekly podcast. The NHA also offers exciting WFPB travel adventures across the globe. Learn more about Wanda and the NHA at www.HealthScience.org.

Karen Ranzi

Karen has followed her passion as a raw vegan health coach since 1998. She is an author, internationally acclaimed speaker, and founder of the online 100-hour Vegan Certification Course for aspiring vegan and raw food health coaches. She is a trained speech and language pathologist of forty-three years. Karen has published four award-winning books and eight eBooks focused on healthy, plant-based, and raw vegan living. Karen's health coaching specializes in helping women with weight, hormonal, and gut issues and raising healthy vegan children. Karen has traveled throughout the United States and abroad to speak on the benefits of a low-fat raw vegan lifestyle. She is the recipient of the Living Now Award in the category of Health and Nutrition, and the Peer-to-Peer Award for Service to Children's Health. Learn more about Karen at www.feelfabulouswithfood.com.

Karin Wentworth-Ping

Based in Sydney, Australia, Karin is a healthy vegan (since 1988) who turned her commitment to veganism into her work as a nutrition coach at Full on Plants Coaching. She offers food and nutrition coaching for people transitioning to a vegan/plant-based diet. Respectful that the process of change is rarely smooth and without obstacles, Karin understands the very personal nature of individual transition and the challenges it poses. With her extensive career as a hypnotherapist and as a personal coach in the corporate sector, she helps clients create a clearly defined personal outcome, plan of action, and readiness to meet challenges and develop new habits and mindsets. She offers coaching for individuals and couples, as well as corporate wellness training. In addition, she provides support and guidance to vegans as a vegan mentor. Learn more about Karin and her work at fullonplantscoaching.com.au.

RESOURCES FOR THRIVING WITH A VEGAN LIFESTYLE

The path to a plant-based lifestyle is often a journey, with many influences and teachers along the way. The following are books and other resources that you may find helpful in the process of adopting, sustaining, and thriving with a plant-powered, vegan lifestyle.

Books

Physical Health

Barnard, Neal D. *Dr. Neal Barnard's Program for Reversing Diabetes: The Scientifically Proven System for Reversing Diabetes without Drugs*. New York: Rodale, 2017.

Barnard, Neal D. *Power Foods for the Brain: An Effective 3-Step Plan to Protect Your Mind and Strengthen Your Memory*. New York: Grand Central Publishing, 2013.

Barnard, Neal D. *Your Body in Balance: The New Science of Food, Hormones, and Health*. New York: Hachette Book Group, 2020.

Bulsiewicz, Will. *Fiber Fueled: The Plant-Based Gut Health Program for Losing Weight, Restoring Your Health, and Optimizing Your Microbiome*. New York: Penguin Random House, 2020.

Campbell, T. Colin, and Thomas M. Campbell II. *The China Study: The Most Comprehensive Study of Nutrition Ever Conducted and the Startling Implications for Diet, Weight Loss, and Long-Term Health*. Dallas: BenBella Books, 2006.

Carr, Kris. *Crazy Sexy Diet: Eat Your Veggies, Ignite Your Spark, and Live Like You Mean It*. Guilford, CT: Skirt!, 2011.

Davis, Garth, with Howard Jacobson. *Proteinaholic: How Our Obsession with Meat Is Killing Us and What We Can Do About It*. New York: HarperCollins, 2015.

Esselstyn, Caldwell B., Jr. *Prevent and Reverse Heart Disease: The Revolutionary, Scientifically Proven, Nutrition-Based Cure*. New York: Penguin Group, 2007.

Fuhrman, Joel. *Eat for Life: The Breakthrough Nutrient-Rich Program for Longevity, Disease Reversal, and Sustained Weight Loss*. New York: HarperOne, 2020.

Fuhrman, Joel. *Eat to Live: The Amazing Nutrient-Rich Program for Fast and Sustained Weight Loss*. New York: Little, Brown & Co., 2011.

Fuhrman, Joel. *Super Immunity: The Essential Nutrition Guide for Boosting Your Body's Defenses to Live Longer, Stronger, and Disease Free*. New York: HarperOne, 2011.

Goldner, Brooke. *Goodbye Autoimmune Disease: How to Prevent and Reverse Chronic Illness and Inflammatory Symptoms Using Supermarket Foods*. Austin, TX: Express Results, 2019.

Goldner, Brooke. *Goodbye Lupus: How a Medical Doctor Healed Herself Naturally with Supermarket Foods*. Austin, TX: Express Results, 2015.

Greger, Michael, with Gene Stone. *How Not to Die: Discover the Foods Scientifically Proven to Prevent and Reverse Disease*. New York: Flatiron Books, 2015.

Lipsky, Sally. *Beyond Cancer: The Powerful Effect of Plant-Based Eating*. Montreal, Canada: Wellness Ink, 2018.

Ornish, Dean, and Anne Ornish. *Undo It: How Simple Lifestyle Change Can Reverse Most Chronic Diseases*. New York: Ballantine Books, 2019.

Robbins, John. *Healthy at 100: How You Can—At Any Age—Dramatically Increase Your Life Span and Your Health Span*. New York: Ballantine Books, 2006.

Sherzai, Dean, and Ayesha Sherzai. *The Alzheimer's Solution: A Breakthrough Program to Prevent and Reverse the Symptoms of Cognitive Decline at Every Age*. New York: HarperCollins, 2017.

Ethics

Baur, Gene. *Farm Sanctuary: Changing Hearts and Minds about Animals and Food*. New York: Touchstone, 2008.

Eisnitz, Gail. *Slaughterhouse: The Shocking Story of Greed, Neglect, and Inhumane Treatment Inside the U.S. Meat Industry*. New York: Prometheus Books, 2007.

Ferdowsian, Hope. *Phoenix Zones: Where Strength Is Born and Resilience Lives*. Chicago: University of Chicago Press, 2018.

Foer, Jonathan Safran. *Eating Animals*. New York: Little, Brown and Co., 2009.

Francione, Gary. *Why Veganism Matters: The Moral Value of Animals*. New York: Columbia University Press, 2020.

Joy, Melanie. *Why We Love Dogs, Eat Pigs, and Wear Cows: An Introduction to Carnism*. San Francisco, CA: Conari Press, 2010.

Kemmerer, Lisa. *Vegan Ethics: AMORE—Five Reasons to Choose Vegan*. VeganTapestry, 2022.

Robbins, John. *Diet for a New America: How Your Food Choices Affect Your Health, Happiness, and the Future of Life on Earth*. Tiburon, CA: HJ Kramer, 1987.

Robbins, John. *The Food Revolution: How Your Diet Can Help Save Your Life and Our World*. San Francisco, CA: Conari Press, 2001.

Scully, Matthew. *Dominion: The Power of Man, the Suffering of Animals, and the Call to Mercy*. New York: St. Martin's Press, 2002.

Sinclair, Todd. *Rebel Vegan Life: A Radical Take on Veganism for a Brave New World*. London: Intrepid Fox, 2021.

Singer, Peter. *Animal Liberation*. New York: Random House, 1990.

Tuttle, Will. *The World Peace Diet: Eating for Spiritual Health and Social Harmony*. Tenth Anniversary ed. New York: Lantern Books, 2016.

Environment

Lyman, Howard F., with Glen Merzer. *Mad Cowboy: Plain Truth from the Cattle Rancher Who Won't Eat Meat*. New York: Scribner, 1998.

Merzer, Glen. *Food Is Climate: A Response to Al Gore, Bill Gates, Paul Hawken, and the Conventional Narrative on Climate Change*. Atlanta, GA: Vivid Thoughts Press, 2021.

Piper, Ashlee. *Give a Sh*t: Do Good, Live Better, Save the Planet*. New York: Running Press, 2018.

Zacharias, Nil, and Gene Stone. *Eat for the Planet: Save the World One Bite at a Time*. New York: Abrams, 2018.

Spirituality and Mindfulness

Adams, Carol J. *The Inner Art of Vegetarianism: Spiritual Practices for Body and Soul*. New York: Lantern Books, 2000.

Blue, Sersie, and Gigi Carter. *Daniel Fast: Why You Should Only Do It Once*. Tustin, CA: Trilogy Christian Publishers, 2023.

Gannon, Sharon. *Yoga & Veganism: The Diet of Enlightenment*. Revised ed. San Rafael, CA: MandalaEarth, 2020.

Moran, Victoria. *The Good Karma Diet: Eat Gently, Feel Amazing, Age in Slow Motion*. New York: Penguin Random House, 2015.

Muelrath, Lani. *The Mindful Vegan: A 30-Day Plan for Finding Health, Balance, Peace, and Happiness*. Dallas, TX: BenBella Books, 2017.

Fitness

Brazier, Brendan. *Thrive: The Vegan Nutrition Guide to Optimal Performance in Sports and Life*. Cambridge, MA: Da Capo Press, 2007.

Cheeke, Robert. *Vegan Bodybuilding and Fitness: The Complete Guide to Building Your Body on a Plant-Based Diet*. Summertown, TN: Healthy Living Publications, 2010.

Esselstyn, Rip. *The Engine 2 Diet: The Texas Firefighter's 28-Day Save-Your-Life Plan that Lowers Cholesterol and Burns Away the Pounds*. New York: Wellness Central, 2009.

Frazier, Matt, and Robert Cheeke. *The Plant Based Athlete: A Game-Changing Approach to Peak Performance*. New York: HarperCollins, 2021.

Healing Food Addictions

Chef A.J., with Glen Merzer. *The Secrets to Ultimate Weight Loss: A Revolutionary Approach to Conquer Cravings, Overcome Food Addiction, and Lose Weight Without Going Hungry.* Hail to the Kale Publishing, 2018.

Giudicelli, Bobbi. *Freedom from a Toxic Relationship with Food: A Journey That Will Give You Your Life Back.* Grass Valley, CA: Let's Tell Your Story Publishing, 2021.

Lisle, Douglas J., and Alan Goldhamer. *The Pleasure Trap: Mastering the Hidden Force that Undermines Health and Happiness.* Summertown, TN: Healthy Living Publications, 2003.

Moran, Victoria. *The Love Powered Diet: Eating for Freedom, Health, and Joy.* New York: Lantern Books, 2009.

Pandemics

Greger, Michael. *How to Survive a Pandemic.* New York: Flatiron Books, 2020.

How Do I Move Toward a Plant-Powered Lifestyle?

Barnard, Neal, D. *The Vegan Starter Kit: Everything You Need to Know About Plant-Based Eating.* New York: Hachette Book Group, 2018.

Day, Jackie. *The Vegan Way: 21 Days to a Happier, Healthier Plant-Based Lifestyle That Will Transform Your Home, Your Diet, and You.* New York: St. Martin's Press, 2016.

Harter, Stephanie. *The Skinny on Eating Like You Give a Damn: How to Embrace a Plant-Based Diet, Combat Injustice, and Be a Rebel for Compassion One Bite at a Time.* Largo, FL: Kewl Publishing, 2019.

McQuirter, Tracye Lynn. *By Any Greens Necessary: A Revolutionary Guide for Black Women Who Want to Eat Great, Get Healthy, Lose Weight, and Look Phat.* Chicago: Lawrence Hill Books, 2010.

Moran, Victoria, with Adair Moran. *Main Street Vegan: Everything You Need to Know to Eat Healthfully and Live Compassionately in the Real World.* New York: Penguin, 2012.

Patrick-Goudreau, Colleen. *The 30-Day Vegan Challenge: The Ultimate Guide to Eating Cleaner, Getting Leaner, and Living Compassionately.* New York: Ballantine Books, 2011.

Silverstone, Alicia. *The Kind Diet: A Simple Guide to Feeling Great, Losing Weight, and Saving the Planet.* New York: Rodale, 2009.

Sinclair, Todd. *Rebel Vegan Life: A Plant-Based Nutrition & Beginner's Guide.* London: Intrepid Fox, 2021.

Singer, Jasmine, and VegNews Magazine. *The VegNews Guide to Being a Fabulous Vegan: Look Good, Feel Good, & Do Good in 30 Days.* New York: Hachette Book Group, 2020.

Taylor, Sarah. *Vegetarian to Vegan: Give Up Dairy. Give Up Eggs. For Good.* Gig Harbor, WA: The Vegan Next Door, 2013.

Nutritional Guidance for a Plant-Based Diet

Davis, Brenda, and Vesanto Melina. *Becoming Vegan: The Complete Guide to Adopting a Healthy, Plant-Based Diet*. Summertown, TN: Book Publishing Co., 2000.

Davis, Brenda, and Vesanto Melina, with Rynn Berry. *Becoming Raw: The Essential Guide to Raw Vegan Diets*. Summertown, TN: Book Publishing Co., 2010.

Davis, Brenda, Vesanto Melina, and Corey Davis. *Plant-Powered Protein: Nutrition Essentials and Dietary Guidelines for All Ages*. Summertown, TN: Healthy Living Publications, 2023.

Hever, Julieanna. *The Complete Idiot's Guide to Plant-Based Nutrition*. New York: Alpha Books, 2011.

Kassam, Shireen, and Zahra Kassam. *Eating Plant-Based: Scientific Answers to Your Nutrition Questions*. London: Hammersmith Books, 2022.

Melina, Vesanto, and Brenda Davis. *The New Becoming Vegetarian: The Essential Guide to a Healthy Vegetarian Diet*. Summertown, TN: Healthy Living Publications, 2003.

Messina, Virginia, with JL Fields. *Vegan for Her: The Woman's Guide to Being Healthy and Fit on a Plant-Based Diet*. Boston, MA: Da Capo Press, 2013.

Norris, Jack, and Virginia Messina. *Vegan for Life: Everything You Need to Know to Be Healthy and Fit on a Plant-Based Diet*. Boston, MA: Da Capo Press, 2011.

Shah, Reshma, and Brenda Davis. *Nourish: The Definitive Plant-Based Nutrition Guide for Families*. Boca Raton, FL: Health Communications, Inc., 2020.

Thriving Emotionally and Socially as a Vegan

Adams, Carol J. *Living Among Meat Eaters: The Vegetarian's Survival Handbook*. New York: Three Rivers Press, 2001.

Baur, Gene, with Gene Stone. *Living the Farm Sanctuary Life: The Ultimate Guide to Eating Mindfully, Living Longer, and Feeling Better Every Day*. New York: Rodale, 2015.

Colb, Sherry F. *Mind if I Eat the Cheeseburger? And Other Questions People Ask Vegans*. New York: Lantern Books, 2013.

Freston, Kathy. *Veganist: Lose Weight, Get Healthy, Change the World*. New York: Weinstein Books, 2011.

Harper, A. Breeze, ed. *Sistah Vegan: Black Female Vegans Speak on Food, Identity, Health, and Society*. New York: Lantern Books, 2010.

Joy, Melanie. *Beyond Beliefs: A Guide to Improving Relationships and Communication for Vegans, Vegetarians, and Meat Eaters*. New York: Lantern Books, 2018.

Joy, Melanie. *Getting Relationships Right: How to Build Resilience and Thrive in Life, Love, and Work*. Oakland, CA: Berrett-Koehler Publishers, 2020.

Kong, Joanne, ed. *Vegan Voices: Essays by Inspiring Changemakers*. New York: Lantern Publishing & Media, 2021.

Lindstrom, Eric C. *The Skeptical Vegan: My Journey from Notorious Meat Eater to Tofu-Munching Vegan—A Survival Guide*. New York: Skyhorse, 2017.

Mann, Clare. *Vystopia: The Anguish of Being Vegan in a Non-Vegan World*. Sydney, Australia: Communicate31, 2018.

Patrick-Goudreau, Colleen. *The Joyful Vegan: How to Stay Vegan in a World That Wants You to Eat Meat, Dairy, and Eggs*. Dallas, TX: BenBella Books, 2019.

Patrick-Goudreau, Colleen. *Vegan's Daily Companion: 365 Days of Inspiration for Cooking, Eating, and Living Compassionately*. Beverly, MA: Quarry Books, 2011.

Sinclair, Todd. *Rebel Vegan Travel Guide: Veganism on the Go*. London: Intrepid Fox, 2021.

Cookbooks

Bodrug, Carleigh. *PlantYou: 140+ Ridiculously Easy, Amazingly Delicious Plant-Based, Oil-Free Recipes*. New York: Hachette Book Group, 2022.

Bulsiewicz, Will. *The Fiber Fueled Cookbook: Inspiring Plant-Based Recipes to Turbocharge Your Health*. New York: Penguin Random House, 2022.

Coscarelli, Chloe. *Chloe's Kitchen: 125 Easy, Delicious Recipes for Making the Food You Love the Vegan Way*. New York: Simon & Schuster, 2012.

Fuhrman, Joel. *Eat to Live Cookbook: 200 Delicious Nutrient Rich Recipes for Fast and Sustained Weight Loss, Reversing Disease, and Lifelong Health*. New York: HarperCollins, 2013.

Greger, Michael, with Gene Stone. *How Not to Die Cookbook: 100+ Recipes to Help Prevent and Reverse Disease*. New York: Flatiron Books, 2017.

Jones, Ellen Jaffe. *Eat Vegan on $4 a Day: A Game Plan for the Budget Conscious Cook*. Summertown, TN: Book Publishing Co., 2011.

Merzer, Glen, with Tracy Childs. *America Goes Vegan: America's Favorite Comfort Foods Made Healthy*. Atlanta, GA: Vivid Thoughts Press, 2023.

Moran, Victoria, and J.L. Fields, with Main Street Vegan Coaches. *The Main Street Vegan Academy Cookbook: Over 100 Plant-Sourced Recipes Plus Practical Tips for the Healthiest, Most Compassionate You*. Dallas: BenBella Books, 2017.

Moskowitz, Isa Chandra. *Vegan with a Vengeance: Over 150 Delicious, Cheap, Animal-Free Recipes that Rock*. New York: Marlowe & Company, 2005.

Okamoto, Toni. *Plant-Based on a Budget: Delicious Vegan Recipes for Under $30 a Week, in Less Than 30 Minutes a Meal*. Dallas: BenBella Books, 2019.

Patrick-Goudreau, Colleen. *The Joy of Vegan Baking: More than 150 Traditional Treats & Sinful Sweets*. Beverly, MA: Fair Winds Press, 2007.

Robertson, Robin. *Vegan Planet: 400 Irresistible Recipes with Fantastic Flavors from Home and Around the World*. Boston: Harvard Common Press, 2003.

Sroufe, Del. *Forks Over Knives—The Cookbook: Over 300 Recipes for Plant-Based Eating All Through the Year*. New York: The Experiment, 2012.

Timberlake, Priscilla, and Lewis Freedman. *The Great Life Cookbook: Whole-food, Vegan, Gluten-Free Meals for Large Gatherings.* 2nd ed. Brooktondale, New York: Coddington Valley Publishing, 2013.

Wenz, Dianne. *Eating Vegan: A Plant-Based Cookbook for Beginners.* Emeryville, CA: Rockridge Press, 2020.

Wenz, Dianne. *The Big Book of Vegan Cooking: 175 Recipes for a Healthy Vegan Lifestyle.* Emeryville. CA: Rockridge Press, 2021.

Wenz, Dianne. *Truly Healthy Vegan Cookbook: 90 Whole-Food Recipes with Deliciously Simple Ingredients.* Emeryville. CA: Rockridge Press, 2019.

Organizations and Websites

American College of Lifestyle Medicine (ACLM), https://lifestylemedicine.org/. Medical society for healthcare professionals dedicated to lifestyle medicine.

American Vegan Society, https://americanvegan.org/. Information, education, and events for promoting a vegan lifestyle.

A Well-Fed World, https://awellfedworld.org/. Plant-based solutions for international hunger relief and environmental sustainability.

The Beet, https://thebeet.com/. Articles on all aspects of plant-based living.

Center for Nutrition Studies, https://nutritionstudies.org/. Recipes, resources, and research.

Christian Vegetarian Association, https://christianveg.org/. Advocates a plant-based diet to reflect Christian values of concern and compassion for all beings.

Climate Healers, https://climatehealers.org/. Information and resources about climate healing.

Coalition for Healthy School Food, https://healthyschoolfood.org/wp/. Promotes plant-based foods and nutrition information in schools.

Daily Dozen App, https://nutritionfacts.org/daily-dozen/. Nutritional tracking app from Dr. Michael Greger.

Farm Animal Rights Movement (FARM), https://farmusa.org/. Advocates for animal rights, veganism, and sustainability.

Farm Sanctuary, https://www.farmsanctuary.org/. Rescue, education, and advocacy to fight the harmful effects of animal agriculture on animals, humans, and the environment.

Food Revolution Network, https://foodrevolution.org/. Articles about plant-based lifestyle and nutrition.

Forks Over Knives, https://www.forksoverknives.com/. Recipes and meal planning.

Gentle World, https://gentleworld.org/. Information and resources for vegan living.

Happy Cow, https://www.happycow.net/. Find vegan and veg-friendly restaurants.

How Do I Go Vegan, https://www.howdoigovegan.com/. Gives information about the reasons for a vegan lifestyle, as well as tips and guidance for going vegan.

Humane Society of the United States (HSUS), https://www.humanesociety.org/all-our-fights. Advocates for animal rights and welfare.

In Defense of Animals (IDA), https://www.idausa.org/. Advocates to protect animals, humans, and the environment from abuse and exploitation.

Institute for Humane Education, https://humaneeducation.org/. Offers programs that teach the connections between human rights, animal protection, and environmental sustainability.

Jewish Veg, https://jewishveg.org/. Educates and promotes a plant-based lifestyle, centered on Jewish values and community.

Living with Harmony, https://livingwithharmony.org/. Information for healing our planet.

Main Street Vegan, https://mainstreetvegan.com/. Blog and podcast about vegan living and a certification and training program for vegan coaches, educators, and entrepreneurs.

Mercy For Animals, https://mercyforanimals.org/. Advocates for animal rights and welfare.

National Health Association (NHA), https://www.healthscience.org/. Promotes benefits of a whole-food, vegan lifestyle, offering a magazine, podcast, and newsletter, as well as educational conferences and travel opportunities.

New Roots Institute, https://www.newrootsinstitute.org/. Empowering the next generation to end factory farming. (Formerly called Factory Farming Awareness Coalition).

No Meat Athlete, https://www.nomeatathlete.com/. Support for athletes to thrive with a plant-based diet.

Nutrition Facts, https://nutritionfacts.org/. Videos and articles reviewing the research on diet, nutrition, and health, shared by Dr. Michael Greger.

Peace Advocacy Network (PAN), https://peaceadvocacynetwork.org/. Promotes a peaceful lifestyle through vegan living. Offers mentoring, education, and support.

People for the Ethical Treatment of Animals (PETA), https://www.peta.org/. Advocates for animal rights and protection.

Physicians Committee for Responsible Medicine (PCRM), https://www.pcrm.org/. Promotes plant-based nutrition and ethical research methods. Offers 21-Day Vegan Kickstart.

Plant-Based Docs, https://plantbaseddocs.com/. Find a plant-based healthcare provider.

Plant-Based on a Budget, https://plantbasedonabudget.com/. Resources, recipes, and meal plans.

Rebel Vegan Life, https://rebelveganlife.com/. Tips for plant-based eating, living, and traveling.

Sentient Media, (https://sentientmedia.org/. Articles about ethical and environmental issues associated with animal agriculture.

Unchained TV, https://unchainedtv.com/. Vegan and plant-based news network.

United in Heart, https://unitedinheart.org/. Solve climate change through coordinated action.

Vegan Health, https://veganhealth.org/. Evidence-based nutrient recommendations for vegans.

Vegan Outreach, https://veganoutreach.org/. Support, mentoring, and nutritional guidance for going vegan.

Vegan Street, https://www.veganstreet.com/. Tips on vegan living, recipes, and community.

Vegan Summerfest, https://summerfest.navs-online.org/. Yearly vegan festival with educational presentations, social events, and delicious vegan food.

Vegetarian Resource Group (VRG), https://www.vrg.org/. Information about all aspects of vegan and vegetarian living.

VegNews, https://vegnews.com/. Recipes and articles from *VegNews* magazine.

Documentaries

A Prayer For Compassion, http://aprayerforcompassion.com/. Highlights how an ethic of compassion for all sentient beings is consistent with spiritual and religious teachings.

Code Blue, https://www.codebluedoc.com/. Reveals problems with the current state of medicine and shows the benefits of a lifestyle medicine approach.

Cowspiracy, https://www.cowspiracy.com/. Shows impact of food choices on the environment.

Dominion, https://www.dominionmovement.com/watch. Australian-based documentary raising awareness of animal exploitation through various industries.

Earthlings, http://www.nationearth.com/. Narrated by Joaquin Phoenix, with music by Moby. Raises awareness of various forms of animal exploitation and their devastating impact.

Eating Our Way to Extinction, https://www.eating2extinction.com/the-movie/. Highlights the dramatic power of our food choices in impacting our environment and ecosystems.

Eating You Alive, https://www.eatingyoualive.com/. A scientific look at the impact of food on our health, and how we can take charge of it through our nutritional choices.

Fat, Sick, and Nearly Dead. https://www.rebootwithjoe.com/joes-films/. Shares the story of Joe Cross, who undergoes a juice fast to reclaim his health, lose weight, and inspire others.

Food, Inc. https://watchdocumentaries.com/food-inc/. Unveils practices of the American food industry, revealing the environmental and ethical impacts of modern animal agriculture.

Forks Over Knives, https://www.forksoverknives.com/the-film/. Landmark documentary showing the healing power of a whole-food, plant-based lifestyle.

Game Changers, https://gamechangersmovie.com/. Engaging film about elite athletes who embrace a plant-based lifestyle, with great benefits for their health and athleticism.

Peaceable Kingdom, https://www.peaceablekingdomfilm.org/. Powerful story of awakening to a new understanding of our relationships with animals.

Plant Pure Nation, https://www.plantpurenation.com/pages/plantpure-nation-movie. A community program demonstrates the health benefits of a plant-based lifestyle.

Plantwise, https://www.adventhealth.com/plantwise-documentary. Shares the life-changing and health-promoting benefits of a plant-based lifestyle.

Seaspiracy, https://www.seaspiracy.org/. Shows the devastating impacts of the fishing industry on our oceans and the planet.

The Invisible Vegan, https://vimeo.com/ondemand/theinvisiblevegan. Explores the problems of unhealthy eating patterns in the African American community.

They're Trying to Kill Us, https://www.theyretryingtokillus.com/. Raises awareness of food deserts and issues impacting health and nutrition in the African American community.

Vegucated, https://www.getvegucated.com/. Documents journey of three New Yorkers who adopt a vegan diet.

What the Health, https://www.whatthehealthfilm.com/. Entertaining exploration of the impact of food and nutrition, and the science supporting the benefits of a plant-based diet.

You Are What You Eat: A Twin Experiment, https://www.netflix.com/title/81133260. Shares the journey of identical twins participating in Stanford University's study on the health effects of vegan and omnivore diets.

APPENDIX: EXPRESSIONS OF VEGAN PURPOSE

Many vegans draw on their gifts, skills, passions, experience, and/or expertise to provide plant-based services and products—whether by working for vegan organizations or by creating their own businesses or nonprofits. Their missions center around issues such as human health, animal advocacy, the environment, vegan cuisine, building community, and sometimes all of the above. Learning how other vegans are serving their purpose may inspire you to find your own calling. The following are some examples of the diverse contributions of my vegan research respondents.

Human health and thriving

- Providing plant-based health, nutrition, and/or fitness coaching
- Doctors whose medical practices center around plant-based nutrition and healthy lifestyle
- Working with organizations that raise awareness of the benefits of plant-based nutrition for various populations—for overall health, as well as preventing or reversing disease
- Writing books or articles about personal healing and/or the science of plant-based nutrition
- Competing in bodybuilding and other types of fitness competitions as a vegan athlete
- Holistic, mind-body-spirit wellness programs incorporating vegan principles

Vegan cuisine

- Vegan chefs, caterers, or culinary educators
- Teaching cooking classes online or in local community

- Opening a vegan restaurant, food stall, or food truck
- Vegan hospitality consultants, helping restaurants increase appealing vegan menu options
- Creating cookbooks, recipes, and/or food blogs
- Veganic gardening (using organic, non-animal-sourced soil conditioners and fertilizers)
- Working for companies that create vegan foods or supplements
- Sharing enticing vegan food at social gatherings or work events

Animal advocacy

- Working for animal protection and advocacy organizations
- Volunteering with animal sanctuaries
- Writing articles or social media posts
- Speaking on podcasts or other programs
- Raising awareness through artwork, books, magazines, or videos
- Participating with activist groups to protest animal harm, cruelty, and exploitation

Environment and climate

- Consulting, teaching, speaking, or writing about the connection between animal agriculture and environmental degradation
- Participating in climate or environmental organizations

Health and food equity

- Involvement in organizations that research and address health disparities among minorities or underserved communities
- Working in the field of humane education, which teaches about the connections between human rights, animal protection, and environmental sustainability, and nurtures students' creative, systems-based, and solution-focused thinking skills
- Participating in plant-based food relief programs

Building community

- Participating in local plant-based or vegan groups
- Organizing a vegan meet-up group
- Organizing or participating in Veg Fests
- Participating with global vegan organizations
- Being involved in summits, conferences, and other events

Vegan services

- Marketing, copywriting, consulting, training, or other services for vegan businesses and organizations
- Mentoring new vegans to successfully transition to and sustain a vegan lifestyle
- Coaching or psychotherapy to support vegans in thriving emotionally and interpersonally
- Vegan support groups
- Financial investing in vegan businesses and companies

NOTES

Introduction

1   *Merriam-Webster's Collegiate Dictionary*, 10th ed. (Springfield, MA: Merriam-Webster, 2001), 1249.

2   Matthew McGough et al., "How Does Health Care Spending in the U.S. Compare to Other Countries?", Peterson-KFF Health System Tracker, February 9, 2023, https://www.healthsystemtracker.org/chart-collection/health-spending-u-s-compare-countries/.

3   "Life Expectancy at Birth, Total Years, All Countries and Economies," The World Bank Data, accessed January 22, 2024, https://data.worldbank.org/indicator/SP.DYN.LE00.IN.

4   Some sources suggest that vegans represent about 3 percent of the US population: Kim Hemi, "Is Veganism Becoming More Popular? Using Data to Track the Growing Trend," *Sentient Media*, May 13, 2022, https://sentientmedia.org/increase-in-veganism/; Charles Stahler and Reed Mangels, *The VRG Vegan Journal*, 2022, Issue 4, https://www.vrg.org/journal/vj2022issue4/2022_issue4_how_many.php; and 3 percent of the global population: "An Exploration into Diets Around the World," Ipsos, August 2018, https://www.ipsos.com/sites/default/files/ct/news/documents/2018-09/an_exploration_into_diets_around_the_world.pdf. Some, however, estimate that vegans represent only 1 percent of the global population: Andrew Anthony, "From Fringe to Mainstream: How Millions Got a Taste for Going Vegan," *The Guardian*, October 10, 2021, https://www.theguardian.com/lifeandstyle/2021/oct/10/from-fringe-to-mainstream-how-millions-got-a-taste-for-going-vegan.

Chapter 1: The Transformative Power of a Vegan Lifestyle

1   Colleen Patrick-Goudreau, *The Joyful Vegan: How to Stay Vegan in a World That Wants You to Eat Meat, Dairy, and Eggs* (Dallas, TX: BenBella Books, 2019), 269.

2   Todd Sinclair, *Rebel Vegan Life: A Radical Take on Veganism for a Brave New World* (London: Intrepid Fox, 2021), 144.

3   Michael Greger with Gene Stone, *How Not to Die: Discover the Foods Scientifically Proven to Prevent and Reverse Disease* (New York: Flatiron Books, 2015); T. Colin Campbell

and Thomas M. Campbell, *The China Study: The Most Comprehensive Study of Nutrition Ever Conducted and the Startling Implications for Diet, Weight Loss, and Long-Term Health* (Dallas: BenBella Books, 2006).

4   Dean Sherzai and Ayesha Sherzai, *The Alzheimer's Solution: A Breakthrough Program to Prevent and Reverse the Symptoms of Cognitive Decline at Every Age* (New York: HarperCollins, 2017).

5   Matt Frazier and Robert Cheeke, *The Plant-Based Athlete: A Game-Changing Approach to Peak Performance* (New York: HarperCollins, 2021).

6   Campbell, *The China Study*; Greger, *How Not to Die*; Joel Fuhrman, *Eat for Life: The Breakthrough Nutrient-Rich Program for Longevity, Disease Reversal, and Sustained Weight Loss* (New York: HarperOne, 2020); Will Bulsiewicz, *Fiber-Fueled: The Plant-Based Gut Health Program for Losing Weight, Restoring Your Health, and Optimizing Your Microbiome* (New York: Penguin Random House, 2020).

7   *Forks Over Knives*, https://www.forksoverknives.com/the-film/; *What the Health*, https://www.whatthehealthfilm.com/; *Game Changers*, https://gamechangersmovie.com/.

8   The Humane Society of the United States, "Plant-Based Eating: Good for Animals, the Environment and You," accessed January 23, 2024, https://www.humanesociety.org/resources/plant-based-eating-good-animals-environment-and-you; A Well-Fed World, "Factory Farms," accessed January 23, 2024, https://awellfedworld.org/factory-farms/; Kitty Block, "More Animals than Ever Before—92.2 Billion—Are Used and Killed Each Year for Food," Humane Society of the United States, June 5, 2023, https://www.humanesociety.org/blog/more-animals-ever-922-billion-are-used-and-killed-each-year-food.

9   For more information about Ag-Gag laws, see Animal Legal Defense Fund, "Issue: Ag-Gag Laws," accessed January 23, 2024, https://aldf.org/issue/ag-gag/.

10   For example, see Jacy Reese, "There Is No Such Thing as Humane Meat or Eggs. Stop Kidding Yourself," *The Guardian*, November 16, 2018, https://www.theguardian.com/food/2018/nov/16/theres-no-such-thing-as-humane-meat-or-eggs-stop-kidding-yourself.

11   Humane Society of the United States (HSUS), https://www.humanesociety.org/all-our-fights; People for the Ethical Treatment of Animals (PETA), https://www.peta.org/; John Robbins, *Diet for a New America: How Your Food Choices Affect Your Health, Happiness, and the Future of Life on Earth* (Tiburon, CA: HJ Kramer, 1987); Jonathan Safran Foer, *Eating Animals* (New York: Little, Brown, and Co., 2009).

12   Robert Goodland and Jeff Anhang, "Livestock and Climate Change: What if the Key Actors in Climate Change are Cows, Pigs, and Chickens?" *World Watch Magazine*, November/December 2009, shared on A Well-Fed World, "World Watch Magazine (2009)," accessed January 23, 2024, https://awellfedworld.org/world-watch-magazine/.

13 Glen Merzer, *Food Is Climate: A Response to Al Gore, Bill Gates, Paul Hawken, and the Conventional Narrative on Climate Change* (Atlanta, GA: Vivid Thoughts Press, 2021), 19.

14 Nil Zacharias and Gene Stone, *Eat for the Planet: Save the Planet One Bite at a Time* (New York: Abrams, 2018), 86.

15 Zacharias, *Eat for the Planet*, 108, 112–3.

16 Zacharias, *Eat for the Planet*, 53–69.

17 "Can Factory Farming Feed the World? The Numbers Say No," *Compassion in World Farming* (blog), August 24, 2017, https://www.ciwf.com/blog/2017/08/can-factory-farming-feed-the-world.

18 Frances Moore Lappe, *Diet for a Small Planet, 10th Anniversary ed.* (New York: Ballantine Books, 1982), 69.

19 "Can Factory Farming Feed the World? The Numbers Say No," *CIWF*, 2017.

20 Zacharias, *Eat for the Planet*, 33–51.

21 Zacharias, *Eat for the Planet*, 89–101.

22 Clara Dell, "What Fish Farming Really Means for the Environment, Animals, and People," *Sentient Media*, November 28, 2023, https://sentientmedia.org/fish-farming/.

23 Zacharias, *Eat for the Planet*, 69.

24 *Cowspiracy*, https://www.cowspiracy.com/; *Seaspiracy*, https://www.seaspiracy.org/; *Eating Our Way to Extinction*, https://www.eating2extinction.com/the-movie/.

25 Zacharias, *Eat for the Planet*; Merzer, *Food Is Climate*.

26 Worldometers, COVID-19 Coronavirus Pandemic, last updated January 22, 2024, https://www.worldometers.info/coronavirus/.

27 Brian L. Pike et al., "The Origin and Prevention of Pandemics," *Clin Infect Dis* 50, no. 12 (June 15, 2010):1636–40, https://doi.org:10.1086/652860, https://www.ncbi.nlm.nih.gov/pmc/articles/PMC2874076/; Michael Greger, "Pandemics: History & Prevention," NutritionFacts.org, March 27, 2020, https://nutritionfacts.org/video/pandemics-history-prevention/; Michael Greger, "Where Do Deadly Coronaviruses Like MERS-CoV Come From?", June 1, 2020, https://nutrition-facts.org/video/where-do-deadly-coronaviruses-like-mers-cov-come-from/.

28 Hyunju Kim et al., "Plant-Based Diets, Pescatarian Diets and COVID-19 Severity: A Population-Based Case-Control Study in Six Countries," *BMJ Nutrition, Prevention & Health* 4, no. 1 (June 2021), https://doi.org:10.1136/bmjnph-2021-000272.

29 Julio Cesar Acosta-Navarro et al., "Vegetarian and Plant-Based Diets Associated with Lower Incidence of COVID-19, *BMJ Nutrition, Prevention & Health*, e000629, 2024, https://doi.org/10.1136/bmjnph-2023-000629.

30 Theresa "Sam" Houghton, "How Does Nutrition Affect the Immune System?" T. Colin Campbell Center for Nutrition Studies, March 20, 2020, https://nutritionstudies.org/how-does-nutrition-affect-the-immune-system/.

31 Michael Greger, *How to Survive a Pandemic* (New York: Flatiron Books, 2020).

32 NutritionFacts.org provides articles and videos covering the latest research on diet, nutrition, and health. For example, this article about pandemics: Michael Greger, "How to Prevent the Next Pandemic," NutritionFacts.org, July 27, 2020, https://nutritionfacts.org/video/how-to-prevent-the-next-pandemic/.

33 *Wikipedia*, definition of "Ahimsa," https://en.wikipedia.org/wiki/Ahimsa.

34 Matilde Nunez del Prado Alanes, "What Is Factory Farming and Why Is it Bad?" *Sentient Media*, October 28, 2022, https://sentientmedia.org/factory-farms/.

35 References to the "cow in the room": Phoebe Weston and Jonathon Watts, "The Cow in the Room: Why Is No One Talking About Farming at COP-26?", *The Guardian*, November 9, 2021, https://www.theguardian.com/environment/2021/nov/09/the-cow-in-the-room-why-is-no-one-talking-about-farming-at-cop26-aoe; Climate Healers website, https://climatehealers.org/.

36 Victoria Moran, with Adair Moran, *Main Street Vegan: Everything You Need to Know to Eat Healthfully and Live Compassionately in the Real World* (New York, Penguin, 2012), 369–370; Jennie Richards, "Albert Einstein Said 'Man Was Not Born to Be a Carnivore,'" Humane Decisions, March 1, 2017, https://www.humanedecisions.com/albert-einstein-said-man-was-not-born-to-be-a-carnivore/.

37 "Definition of Veganism," The Vegan Society, accessed January 22, 2024, https://www.vegansociety.com/go-vegan/definition-veganism.

Chapter 2: The Courage to Live Your Values

1 Avi Solomon, "Working Undercover in a Slaughterhouse: An Interview with Timothy Pachirat," *Medium.com*, August 25, 2014, https://medium.com/learning-for-life/working-undercover-in-a-slaughterhouse-an-interview-with-timothy-pachirat-c6d7f37eef9c.

2 Michael Greger, with Gene Stone, *How Not to Die: Discover the Foods Scientifically Proven to Prevent and Reverse Disease* (New York: Flatiron Books, 2015).

3 Sections of this story about my vegan awakening were shared in my blog article: Angela Crawford, "How Veganism Inspired Me to Find My Voice," October 7, 2020, https://angelacrawfordphd.com/2020/10/07/how-veganism-inspired-me-to-find-my-voice/.

4 Leon Festinger, *A Theory of Cognitive Dissonance* (Evanston, IL: Row, Peterson, & Co., 1957); Jennifer Tzeses, "Tell Me Everything I Need to Know About Cognitive Dissonance," Health Central, October 30, 2020, https://www.healthcentral.com/mental-health/cognitive-dissonance.

5 Kristina Zagame, "Pet Spending Trends of 2024: Older Americans Spend More on Pets," Market Watch Guides, updated January 11, 2024, https://www.marketwatch.com/guides/insurance-services/pet-spending-trends/.

6   Nico Pitney, "Revolution on the Animal Farm," *HuffPost*, updated September 23, 2016, https://www.huffpost.com/entry/farm-animal-rights-revolution_n_577304f6e4b0352fed3e5b16.

7   Colleen Patrick-Goudreau, *The Joyful Vegan: How to Stay Vegan in a World that Wants You to Eat Meat, Dairy, and Eggs* (Dallas, TX: BenBella Books, 2019), 7.

8   A Well-Fed World, "Factory Farms," https://awellfedworld.org/factory-farms/; Kitty Block, "More Animals than Ever Before-92.2 Billion-Are Used and Killed Each Year for Food," Humane Society of the United States, June 5, 2023, https://www.humanesociety.org/blog/more-animals-ever-922-billion-are-used-and-killed-each-year-food.

9   Gretchen Kuck and Gary Schnitkey, "An Overview of Meat Consumption in the United States," Farm Doc Daily, May 12, 2021, https://farmdocdaily.illinois.edu/2021/05/an-overview-of-meat-consumption-in-the-united-states.html.

10   "Meat Supply per Person," Our World in Data, 2020, https://ourworldindata.org/grapher/meat-supply-per-person?tab=table; Jen Flatt Osborn, "The Meat of the Matter: Understanding U.S. Meat Consumption," World Animal Foundation, October 10, 2023, https://worldanimalfoundation.org/advocate/us-meat-consumption/.

11   Hannah Ritchie, Pablo Rosado, and Max Roser, "Meat and Dairy Production," Our World in Data, last updated December 2023, https://ourworldindata.org/meat-production.

12   Pitney, "Revolution on the Animal Farm," *HuffPost*.

13   This is thanks to the courageous undercover work of animal activists, who have dared to witness, photograph, and share the horrific practices in factory farming and slaughterhouses, despite Ag-Gag laws created by the animal agriculture industry to prevent us from seeing this footage. One might wonder why these Ag-Gag laws exist, if not to hide from the public the horror of what really happens, so that we will not speak out or protest.

14   Which animals are considered "edible" differs in different cultures. For example, South Korea's dog meat trade is horrifying to those of us in Western countries. At the time of writing this book, South Korea recently voted to ban dog meat trade, which will be enforced starting in 2027: Koh Ewe, "South Korea's Parliament Unanimously Passes Historic Dog Meat Ban," *Time*, January 9, 2024, https://time.com/6553409/south-korea-passes-dog-meat-trade-ban.

15   Melanie Joy, *Why We Love Dogs, Eat Pigs and Wear Cows: An Introduction to Carnism* (San Francisco, CA: Conari Press, 2010), 27.

16   Joy, *Why We Love Dogs, Eat Pigs, and Wear Cows*, 30.

17   Joy, *Why We Love Dogs, Eat Pigs, and Wear Cows*, 97.

18   Joy, *Why We Love Dogs, Eat Pigs, and Wear Cows*, 95–113.

19   Steve Loughman, Boyka Bratanova, and Elisa Puvia, "The Meat Paradox: How Are We Able to Love Animals and Love Eating Animals?", *In-Mind Italia* 1 (January

2012): 15–18, https://www.researchgate.net/publication/258332248_The_Meat_Paradox_How_are_we_able_to_love_animals_and_love_eating_animals.

20 For example: Rob Percival, *The Meat Paradox: Eating, Empathy, and the Future of Meat* (New York: Pegasus Books, 2022).

21 Steve Loughnan, Brock Bastion, and Nick Haslam, "The Psychology of Eating Animals," *Current Directions in Psychological Science* 23, no. 2 (October 2014): 104–8, https://doi.org/10.1177/0963721414525781.

22 Sarah Gradidge et al., "A Structured Literature Review of the Meat Paradox (Accepted Author Manuscript)," *Social Psychological Bulletin* (August 2021), https://doi.org/10.32872/spb.5953.

23 Winston J. Craig and Anne Reed Mangels, "Position of the American Dietetic Association: Vegetarian Diets," *J Am Diet Assoc.* 109, no. 7 (July 2009): 1266–82, https://doi.org10.1016/j.jada.2009.05.027.

24 Zoe Weil, "Are Manufactured Desires Eclipsing Your Deepest Desires?" *Psychology Today* (November 17, 2022), https://www.psychologytoday.com/us/blog/becoming-solutionary/202211/are-manufactured-desires-eclipsing-your-deepest-values.

25 Researchers Matthew Ruby and colleagues added a 4th N, which they refer to as "Nice." In addition to eating meat because it is "Natural, Normal, and Necessary," we also justify meat eating because it "tastes good." See: Marta Zaraska, "Meet the Meat Paradox," *Scientific American*, July 1, 2016, https://www.scientificamerican.com/article/meet-the-meat-paradox/.

26 Neal D. Barnard, *The Cheese Trap: How Breaking a Surprising Addiction Will Help You Lose Weight, Gain Energy, and Get Healthy* (New York: Hachette Book Group, 2017), 37–53.

27 Michael Moss, *Salt, Sugar, Fat: How the Food Giants Hooked Us* (New York: Random House, 2014); Douglas J. Lisle and Alan Goldhamer, *The Pleasure Trap: Mastering the Hidden Force that Undermines Health and Happiness* (Summertown, TN: Healthy Living Publications, 2003).

28 To learn more about Nancy Arenas, check out her essay, "A Journey to the Awakening of the Body, Mind, and Soul," in *Vegan Voices: Essays by Inspiring Changemakers* (Joanne Kong, ed., New York: Lantern, 2021), 133–7.

29 John Oberg, Instagram, February 2023, https://www.instagram.com/p/CoKdkgFs5ME/?ref=6bgtt2veydyv&hl=af.

Chapter 3: Expand Your Circle of Compassion

1 Some sections of this chapter were also shared in an article I wrote for *Main Street Vegan Academy* blog: Angela Crawford, "Awakening Compassion," April 18, 2023, https://mainstreetvegan.com/awakening-compassion-by-angela-crawford-ph-d-mvlce/.

2 Dacher Keltner, "The Compassionate Species," *Greater Good Magazine*, July 31, 2012, https://greatergood.berkeley.edu/article/item/the_compassionate_species.

3 Charles Darwin, *The Descent of Man* (UK: John Murray, 1871).

4   John Robbins, *Diet for a New America: How Your Food Choices Affect Your Health, Happiness, and the Future of Life on Earth* (Tiburon, CA: HJ Kramer, 1987).

5   *Merriam-Webster's Collegiate Dictionary*, 10th ed. (Springfield, MA: Merriam-Webster, 2001), 378, 234.

6   The Greater Good Science Center at University of California at Berkeley, "What Is Compassion?", *Greater Good Magazine*, accessed January 23, 2024, https://greatergood.berkeley.edu/topic/compassion/definition.

7   Daniel Goleman, *Emotional Intelligence: Why It Can Matter More Than IQ* (New York: Random House, 2012).

8   Amy J. Wilson, *Empathy for Change: How to Create a More Understanding World* (Potomac, MD: New Degree Press, 2021), 34.

9   Karen Armstrong and Archbishop Desmond Tutu, "Compassion Unites the World's Faiths," CNN TED Talk Tuesdays, November 10, 2009, https://www.cnn.com/2009/OPINION/11/10/armstrong.tutu.charter.compassion/index.html.

10 Keltner, "The Compassionate Species," *Greater Good Magazine*.

11 Keltner, "The Compassionate Species." *Greater Good Magazine*.

12 Tania Singer and Olga M. Klimecki, "Empathy and Compassion," *Current Biology* 24, no. 18 (September 2014): R875–R878, https://pubmed.ncbi.nlm.nih.gov/25247366/.

13 Dacher Keltner, *Born to Be Good: The Science of a Meaningful Life* (New York: W.W. Norton & Company, 2009), 6.

14 Singer and Klimecki, "Empathy and Compassion."

15 Singer and Klimecki, "Empathy and Compassion."

16 Tricia Dowling, "Compassion Does Not Fatigue!", *Can Vet J* 59, no. 7 (July 2018): 749–50, https://www.ncbi.nlm.nih.gov/pmc/articles/PMC6005077/.

17 Tara Brach, *Radical Compassion: Learning to Love Yourself and Your World with the Practice of RAIN* (New York: Penguin Random House, 2019), 211–2.

18 Colleen Patrick-Goudreau, *The Joyful Vegan: How to Stay Vegan in a World that Wants You to Eat Meat, Dairy, and Eggs* (Dallas, TX: BenBella Books, 2019), 70.

19 Heather S. Lonczak, "20 Reasons Why Compassion Is So Important in Psychology," Positive Psychology, June 7, 2019, https://positivepsychology.com/why-is-compassion-important/#why-is-compassion-important-and-necessary.

20 Singer and Klimecki, "Empathy and Compassion."

21 "The Link Between Cruelty to Animals and Violence Toward Humans," Animal Legal Defense Fund, https://aldf.org/article/the-link-between-cruelty-to-animals-and-violence-toward-humans-2/.

22 "Child Health & Development," Human Animal Bond Research Institute (HABRI), https://habri.org/research/child-health/.

23 "The Power of Pets: Health Benefits of Human-Animal Interactions," NIH News in Health, February 2018, https://newsinhealth.nih.gov/2018/02/power-pets.

24 To learn more about Farm Sanctuary: https://www.farmsanctuary.org/.

25 "Meet Your Meat," PETA, https://www.peta.org/videos/meet-your-meat/; Erin Janus, "Dairy Is Scary: The Industry Explained in 5 Minutes," YouTube, December 27, 2015, https://www.youtube.com/watch?v=UcN7SGGoCNI.

26 *Vegucated*, https://getvegucated.com/film/; *Peaceable Kingdom*, https://www.peaceablekingdomfilm.org/; *Cowspiracy*, https://www.cowspiracy.com/.

27 *Earthlings*, https://www.nationearth.com/; *Dominion*, https://www.dominionmovement.com/watch.

28 Brach, *Radical Compassion*, xix.

29 To learn more about Anita's story, check out her article in the *Main Street Academy* blog: https://mainstreetvegan.com/returning-to-veganism-a-journey-through-grief-by-anita-sherman-moran-rn-m-s-vlce/.

30 To learn more about Nancy Poznak, check out her essay, "Awakening to Compassion Across the Decades" in *Vegan Voices: Essays by Inspiring Changemakers* (Joanne Kong, ed., New York: Lantern, 2021), 169–74.

31 To find animal sanctuaries in the US and internationally: https://vegan.com/blog/sanctuaries/; https://sanctuaryfederation.org/find-a-sanctuary/.

32 Amanda Knose, "Definition, Techniques, & Benefits," Choosing Therapy, December 6, 2022, https://www.choosingtherapy.com/loving-kindness-meditation/; James N. Kirby, James R. Doby, Nicola Petrocchi, and Paul Gilbert, "The Science of Compassion Training," Awake Academy, accessed on January, 23, 2024, https://www.awakeacademy.org/the-science-of-compassion-training/.

33 My audio recording of this exercise is available at https://angelacrawfordphd.com/meditations/.

Chapter 4: Connect with Deeper Meaning and Purpose

1 Victor E. Frankl, *Man's Search for Meaning* (Boston, MA: Beacon Press, 1959).

2 Laura A. King, Samantha J. Heintzelman, and Sarah J. Ward, "Beyond the Search for Meaning: A Contemporary Science of the Experience of Meaning in Life," *Current Directions in Psychological Science* 25, no. 4, (August 2016): 211–6, https://doi.org/10.1177/0963721416656354.

3 The Greater Good Science Center at University of California at Berkeley, "What Is Purpose?", *Greater Good Magazine*, accessed January 23, 2024, https://greatergood.berkeley.edu/topic/purpose/definition#what-is-purpose.

4 Jeremy Sutton, "15 Ways to Find Your Purpose of Life and Realize Your Meaning," Positive Psychology, October 15, 2020, https://positivepsychology.com/find-your-purpose-of-life/.

5 The Greater Good Science Center at University of California at Berkeley, "Why Pursue It?", *Greater Good Magazine*, accessed January 23, 2024, https://greatergood.berkeley.edu/topic/purpose/definition#why-find-purpose.

Notes

6   Frankl, *Man's Search for Meaning*.

7   Dan Buettner, *The Blue Zones: Lessons for Living Longer from the People Who've Lived the Longest* (Washington D.C.: National Geographic, 2008).

8   Roy F. Baumeister et al., "Some Key Differences Between a Happy Life and a Meaningful Life," *The Journal of Positive Psychology* 8, no. 6 (2013): 505–16.

9   Baumeister et al., "Some Key Differences Between a Happy Life and a Meaningful Life," 512.

10   Tim Kelley, *True Purpose: 12 Strategies for Discovering the Difference You Are Meant to Make* (Berkeley, CA: Transcendent Solutions Press, 2009), 22.

11   Survey respondents were asked, "What led to your decision to become vegan? Check any of the following that impacted your decision: Compassion for animals, Environmental concerns, Health reasons, Improving fitness, Concerns about hunger and food justice, Worker justice, or Other." They were then asked, "What factors have influenced you in staying vegan? Check all that apply." They were given the same list to choose from. For both questions, participants were able to check as many items as they wished. Animal compassion was the most highly endorsed reason for *becoming* vegan (81 percent), followed by health (50 percent) and environmental reasons (46 percent). When asked why they *stayed* vegan, again, animal compassion (92 percent) received the most responses, followed by environmental reasons (80 percent), and health (70 percent). Other reasons cited for staying vegan included concerns about food justice (44 percent), improving fitness (40 percent), and worker justice (35 percent). Respondents tended to list one or two primary reasons for *becoming* vegan, but often endorsed several reasons for *staying* vegan.

12   Phillip Wollen, foreword to *Food Is Climate*, by Glen Merzer (Atlanta, GA: Vivid Thoughts Press, 2021), 14.

13   To learn more about Jacque and her foundation: "Meet Jacque Salomon," Seeds to Inspire Foundation, https://www.seedstoinspire.org/jacque-salomon.

14   I have used the Wise Advisor meditation with clients over the years, created from a synthesis of various guided meditations, though perhaps most strongly influenced by psychologist Laurel Parnell's "Inner Advisor Exercise," *Attachment-Focused EMDR: Healing Relational Trauma* (New York: W.W. Norton & Company, Inc., 2013), 67–8.

15   My audio recording of the Wise Advisor meditation is available at https://angelacrawfordphd.com/meditations/.

Chapter 5: Create Authentic Fulfillment

1   Scott Barry Kaufman, *Transcend: The New Science of Self-Actualization* (New York: Penguin Random House, 2021), xxvi.

2   Christopher Peterson, "What Is Positive Psychology and What Is It Not?", *Psychology Today*, May 16, 2008, https://www.psychologytoday.com/us/blog/the-good-life/200805/what-is-positive-psychology-and-what-is-it-not.

3   Martin E.P. Seligman, *Flourish: A Visionary New Understanding of Happiness and Well-Being* (New York: Free Press, 2011), 19–21.

4   "What Is Happiness?" *Greater Good Magazine*, accessed 1/23/2024 (article quotes Sonja Lyubomirsky's definition of happiness from her book *The How of Happiness*, 2007), https://greatergood.berkeley.edu/topic/happiness/definition.

5   Seligman, *Flourish*, 20.

6   Seligman, *Flourish*, 21.

7   Martin E.P. Seligman, *Authentic Happiness: Using the New Positive Psychology to Realize Your Potential for Lasting Fulfillment* (New York: Free Press, 2002).

8   Seligman, *Flourish*.

9   Barbara L. Frederickson, "The Role of Positive Emotions in Positive Psychology: The Broaden-and-Build Theory of Positive Emotions," *Am Psychol.* 56, no. 3 (March 2001): 218–26, https://doi.org/10.1037//0003-066x.56.3.218.

10   Courtney E. Ackerman, "What Are Positive Emotions in Psychology? (+List & Examples)," Positive Psychology, March 12, 2018, https://positivepsychology.com/positive-emotions-list-examples-definition-psychology/.

11   Jeffrey Adam Smith, "How Much Control Do You Have Over Your Own Happiness?" *Greater Good Magazine*, May 11, 2022, https://greatergood.berkeley.edu/article/item/how_much_control_do_you_have_over_your_own_happiness.

12   "Global Happiness Study: What Makes People Happy Around the World," Ipsos, August 2019, https://www.ipsos.com/sites/default/files/ct/news/documents/2019-08/Happiness-Study-report-August-2019.pdf.

13   Jordi Quoidbach et al., "Emodiversity and the Emotional Ecosystem," *Journal of Experimental Psychology* 143, no. 6 (2014), https://doi:10.1037/a0038025.

14   See discussions of these concepts in: Kendra Cherry, "What Is Happiness? Defining Happiness, and How to Be Happier," Very Well Mind, November 7, 2022,, https://www.verywellmind.com/what-is-happiness-4869755; and Ilona Boniwell, *Positive Psychology in a Nutshell: The Science of Happiness* (Berkshire, England: Open University Press), 2012, 49–58.

15   Doris Baumann and Willibald Ruch, "Measuring What Counts in Life: The Development and Initial Validation of the Fulfilled Life Scale," *Frontiers in Psychology* 12 (January 11, 2022), https://doi.org/10.3389/fpsyg.2021.795931.

16   See Michael Greger, How Not to Die; T. Colin Campbell, *The China Study*.

17   Dean Sherzai and Ayesha Sherzai, *The Alzheimer's Solution* (New York: HarperCollins, 2017).

18   Hayden Stewart and Jeffrey Hyman, "Americans Still Can Meet Fruit and Vegetable Dietary Guidelines for $2.10 - $2.60 Per Day," USDA Economic Research Service, June 3, 2019, https://www.ers.usda.gov/amber-waves/2019/june/americans-still-can-meet-fruit-and-vegetable-dietary-guidelines-for-210-260-per-day/.

Notes

19   Dominika Głąbska et al.. "Fruit and Vegetable Intake and Mental Health in Adults: A Systematic Review," *Nutrients* 12, no. 1 (2020): 115, https://doi.org/10.3390/nu12010115,

20   For example: Neel Ocean et al., "Lettuce Be Happy: A Longitudinal UK Study on the Relationship Between Fruit and Vegetable Consumption and Well-Being," *Social Science & Medicine* 222 (2019): 335–45, https://www.sciencedirect.com/science/article/pii/S0277953618306907; David Blanchflower et al., "Is Psychological Well-Being Linked to the Consumption of Fruit and Vegetables?" National Bureau of Economic Research, NBER Working Paper Series (October 2012), https://www.nber.org/system/files/working_papers/w18469/w18469.pdf; Seanna McMartin et al., "The Association Between Fruit and Vegetable Consumption and Mental Health Disorders: Evidence from Five Waves of a National Survey of Canadians," *Prev Med.* 56, no. 3–4 (March 2013): 225–30, https://doi.org/10.1016/j.ypmed.2012.12.016; Aline Richard et al., "Associations Between Fruit and Vegetable Consumption and Psychological Distress: Results from a Population-Based Study," *BMC Psychiatry* 15, 213 (October 2015), https://doi.org/10.1186/s12888-015-0597-4.

21   Redzo Mujcic, "Are Fruit and Vegetables Good for Our Mental and Physical Health? Panel Data Evidence from Australia," Munich Personal RePEc Archive (MPRA), October 8, 2014, https://mpra.ub.uni-muenchen.de/59149/1/MPRA_paper_59149.pdf; Bonnie White et al., "Many Apples a Day Keep the Blues Away: Daily Experiences of Negative and Positive Affect and Food Consumption in Young Adults. *Br J Health Psychol.* 18, no. 4 (November 2013):782-98, https://doi.org/10.1111/bjhp.12021.

22   Tamlin Conner et al., "On Carrots and Curiosity: Eating Fruit and Vegetables Is Associated with Greater Flourishing in Daily Life," *Br J Health Psychol.* 20, no. 2 (May 2015): 413–27, https://doi.org/10.1111/bjhp.12113.

23   White et al., "Many Apples a Day."

24   Redzo Mujcic and Andrew Oswald, "Evolution of Well-Being and Happiness After Increases in Consumption of Fruit and Vegetables," *American Journal of Public Health* 106, no. 8 (August 2016): 1504–10, https://doi.org/10.2105/AJPH.2016.303260.

25   For example: Uma Naidoo, *This Is Your Brain on Food: An Indispensable Guide to the Surprising Foods that Fight Depression, Anxiety, PTSD, OCD, ADHD, and More* (New York: Little, Brown Spark, 2020).

26   Camille Lassale et al., "Healthy Dietary Indices and Risk of Depressive Outcomes: A Systematic Review and Meta-Analysis of Observational Studies," *Molecular Psychiatry* 24 (2019): 965–86, https://doi.org/10.1038/s41380-018-0237-8; Rachelle S. Opie et al., "A Modified Mediterranean Dietary Intervention for Adults with Major Depression: Dietary Protocol and Feasibility

Data from the SMILES Trial," *Nutr Neurosci.* 21, no. 7 (September 2018): 487–501, https://doi.org/10.1080/1028415X.2017.1312841.

27 Almudena Sanchez-Villegas et al., "Association of the Mediterranean Dietary Pattern with Incidence of Depression," *Arch Gen Psychiatry* 66, no. 10 (2009): 1090–8, https://doi:10.1001/archgenpsychiatry.2009.129; Ujue Fresán et al., "Does the MIND Diet Decrease Depression Risk? A Comparison with Mediterranean Diet in the SUN Cohort," *Eur J Nutr.* 58, no. 3 (April 2019): 1271–82, https://doi.org/10.1007/s00394-018-1653-x.

28 Bonnie L. Beezhold, Carol S. Johnston, and Deanna R. Daigle, "Vegetarian Diets Are Associated with Healthy Mood States: A Cross-Sectional Study in Seventh Day Adventist Adults," *Nutrition Journal* 9, no. 26 (June 2010), https://doi.org/10.1186/1475-2891-9-26.

29 Bonnie Beezhold et al., "Vegans Report Less Stress and Anxiety than Omnivores," *Nutr Neurosci.* 18, no. 7 (October 2015): 289–96, https://doi:10.11 79/1476830514Y.0000000164.

30 Erman Senturk et al., "Is Meat-Free Diet Related to Anxiety, Depression, and Disordered Eating Behaviors? A Cross-Sectional Survey in a Turkish Sample," *Annals of Medical Research* 30, no. 5 (May 2023): 569–75, https://doi.org/10.5455/annalsmedres.2023.01.026.

31 Bonnie L. Beezhold and Carol S. Johnston, "Restriction of Meat, Fish, and Poultry in Omnivores Improves Mood: A Pilot Randomized Controlled Trial. *Nutr J* 11, no. 9 (February 2012), https://doi.org/10.1186/1475-2891-11-9.

32 Ulka Agarwal et al., "A Multicenter Randomized Controlled Trial of a Nutrition Intervention Program in a Multiethnic Adult Population in the Corporate Setting Reduces Depression and Anxiety and Improves Quality of Life: The GEICO Study," *Am J Health Promot.* 29, no. 4 (March–April 2015): 245–54, https://doi.org/10.4278/ajhp.130218-QUAN-72.

33 Julia K. Boehm et al., "Association Between Optimism and Serum Antioxidants in the Midlife in the United States Study. *Psychosom Med.* 75, no. 1 (January 2013): 2–10, https://doi.org/10.1097/PSY.0b013e31827c08a9; May A. Beydoun et al., "Antioxidant Status and Its Association with Elevated Depressive Symptoms among US Adults: National Health and Nutrition Examination Surveys 2005-6," *Br J Nutr.* 109, no. 9 (May 2013): 1714–29, https://doi.org/10.1017/S0007114512003467; Fernando Gomez-Pinilla, and Trang Nguyen, "Natural Mood Foods: The Actions of Polyphenols Against Psychiatric and Cognitive Disorders," *Nutr Neurosci.* 15, no. 3 (May 2012): 127–33, https://doi.org/10.11 79/1476830511Y.0000000035.

34 Megan Edwards, "The No-Nonsense Guide to Antioxidants: Facts and Myths Explained," Forks Over Knives, September 28, 2022, https://www.forksoverknives.com/wellness/no-nonsense-guide-to-antioxidants/.

35   Monica H. Carlsen et al., "The Total Antioxidant Content of More than 3100 Foods, Beverages, Spices, Herbs and Supplements Used Worldwide," *Nutr J* 9, no. 3 (January 2010), https://doi.org/10.1186/1475-2891-9-3.

36   "Understanding Acute and Chronic Inflammation," Harvard Health Publishing, April 1, 2020, https://www.health.harvard.edu/staying-healthy/understanding-acute-and-chronic-inflammation; "What Is Chronic Inflammation?" Harvard Health Publishing, October 1, 2020, https://www.health.harvard.edu/diseases-and-conditions/what-is-chronic-inflammation.

37   Michael Berk et al., "So Depression Is an Inflammatory Disease, But Where Does the Inflammation Come From?" *BMC Med* 11, 200 (September 2013), https://doi.org/10.1186/1741-7015-11-200.

38   Janett Barbaresko et al., "Pattern Analysis and Biomarkers of Low-Grade Inflammation: A Systematic Literature Review." *Nutr Rev.* 71, no. 8 (August 2013): 511–27. https://doi.org/10.1111/nure.12035.

39   Michel Lucas et al., "Inflammatory Dietary Pattern and Risk of Depression Among Women," *Brain Behav Immun* 36 (February 2014): 46–53, https://doi.org/10.1016/j.bbi.2013.09.014,.

40   Hui Xu et al., "Exploration of the Association Between Dietary Fiber Intake and Depressive Symptoms in Adults," *Nutrition* 54 (October 2018): 48–53, https://doi.org/10.1016/j.nut.2018.03.009.

41   Jeremy Appleton, "The Gut-Brain Axis: Influence of Microbiota on Mood and Mental Health," *Integr Med (Encinitas)* 17, no. 4 (August 2018):28-32, https://www.ncbi.nlm.nih.gov/pmc/articles/PMC6469458/.

42   Faezeh Saghafian et al., "Dietary Fiber Intake, Depression, and Anxiety: A Systematic Review and Meta-Analysis of Epidemiologic Studies," *Nutr Neurosci* 26, no. 2 (February 2023): 108–26, https://doi.org/10.1080/1028415X.2021.2020403.

43   Katherine D. McManus, "Should I Be Eating More Fiber?" Harvard Health Publishing, February 27, 2019, https://www.health.harvard.edu/blog/should-i-be-eating-more-fiber-2019022115927.

44   Edwards, "The No-Nonsense Guide to Antioxidants," Forks Over Knives, 2022.

45   A few examples include Avlin Woodward and Gabby Landsverk, "People Who Eat Meat Report Lower Levels of Depression and Anxiety than Vegans Do, A Recent Analysis Suggests," *Business Insider*, October 27, 2021, https://www.businessinsider.com/vegans-report-higher-depression-anxiety-than-meat-eaters-2021-10; "Vegetarians More Likely to Be Depressed Than Meat Eaters," *Neuroscience News*, October 7, 2022, https://neurosciencenews.com/vegetarians-depression-21594/; Jill Waldbieser, "The Scary Mental Health Risks of Going Meatless," *Women's Health*, December 2, 2015, https://www.womenshealthmag.com/food/a19941229/side-effects-of-vegetarianism/.

46 For example, limitations of the above *Women's Health* article are discussed here: Ginny Messina, "Will A Vegetarian Diet Make You Depressed?" *The Vegan RD* (blog), December 30, 2015, https://www.theveganrd.com/2015/12/will-a-vegetarian-diet-make-you-depressed/.

47 Urska Dobersek et al., "Meat and Mental Health: A Systematic Review of Meat Abstention and Depression, Anxiety, and Related Phenomena," *Critical Reviews in Food Science and Nutrition* 61, no. 4 (2021): 622–35, https://www.tandfonline.com/doi/full/10.1080/10408398.2020.1741505; Urska Dobersek et al., "Meat and Mental Health: A Meta-Analysis of Meat Consumption, Depression, and Anxiety," *Critical Reviews in Food Science and Nutrition* 63, no. 19 (2023): 3556–73, https://www.tandfonline.com/doi/full/10.1080/10408398.2021.1974336.

48 Dobersek et al., "Meat and Mental Health: A Systematic Review," 622.

49 Beezhold and Johnston, "Restriction of Meat, Fish, and Poultry in Omnivores Improves Mood."

50 Gabby Landsverk, "There Are Serious Problems with a Widely Shared Study that Claimed Meat Eaters Have Better Mental Health than Vegetarians," *Business Insider*, May 2020, https://www.insider.com/study-does-not-say-meat-eating-improves-mental-health-2020-5.

51 For a discussion of limitations of the Dobersek et al. meta-analysis research, see Joel Kahn, "The Vegan Diet and Depression: What You Need to Know," LiveKindly, accessed January 24, 2024, https://www.livekindly.com/meat-vegan-diet-depression/.

52 Joane Matta et al., "Depressive Symptoms and Vegetarian Diets: Results from the Constances Cohort," *Nutrients* 10, no. 11 (2018): 1695, https://doi.org/10.3390/nu10111695.

53 Kristin Lavallee et al., "Vegetarian Diet and Mental Health: Cross-sectional and Longitudinal Analyses in Culturally Diverse Samples," *J Affect Disord* 1, no. 248 (April 2019): 147–54, https://doi.org/10.1016/j.jad.2019.01.035.

54 Dobersek et al., "Meat and Mental Health: A Systematic Review," 633; Dobersek et al., "Meat and Mental Health: A Meta-Analysis," 3571.

55 Landsverk, "There Are Serious Problems."

56 Unfortunately, the potential of bias in research due to industry funding is far from an infrequent problem. This issue is discussed in depth by Dr. T. Colin Campbell in *The China Study*, Chapter 15, "The 'Science' of the Industry," 289–303. Studies that are funded by prosperous industries such as "Big Ag" or "Big Pharma" raise concerns that conflict of interest may influence researchers' approach, findings, and conclusions.

57 Mohammadreza Askari et al., "Vegetarian Diet and the Risk of Depression, Anxiety, and Stress Symptoms: A Systematic Review and Meta-Analysis of

Observational Studies," *Crit Rev Food Sci Nutr* 62, no. 1 (2022): 261–71, https://doi.org/10.1080/10408398.2020.1814991.

58 This societal orientation toward promoting meat-based diets and denouncing plant-based diets reminds me of times past when doctors who were smokers advocated for the health benefits of cigarette smoking. Of course, we know better now—at least when it comes to the dangers of cigarette smoking.

59 Neal D. Barnard, *Your Body in Balance: The New Science of Food, Hormones, and Health* (New York: Hachette Book Group, 2020), 162–87; Ginny Messina, *Vegan for Her: The Woman's Guide to Being Healthy and Fit on a Plant-Based Diet* (Boston, MA: Da Capo Press, 2013), 217–28; Ginny Messina, "Soyfoods, Olive Oil, Beans, and Omega-3's: A Vegan Plan for Reducing Depression," *The Vegan RD* (blog), September 23, 2015, https://www.theveganrd.com/2015/09/soyfoods-olive-oil-beans-and-omega-3s-a-vegan-plan-for-reducing-depression.

60 While the RDA for Vitamin B-12 is 2.4 mcg daily, some sources recommend higher amounts. Based on recent research that suggests heightened risk of stroke (and other health issues) with suboptimal B-12 levels, Dr. Michael Greger recommends 50 mcg of B-12 daily, or 2000 mcg weekly. Higher doses are recommended for those over age sixty-five. See Michael Greger, "Optimum Nutrient Recommendations," NutritionFacts.org, accessed 9/5/2024, https://nutritionfacts.org/optimum-nutrient-recommendations/.

61 Sunny Fitzgerald, "The Secret to Mindful Travel? A Walk in the Woods," *National Geographic*, October 18, 2019, https://www.nationalgeographic.com/travel/article/forest-bathing-nature-walk-health.

Chapter 6: The Power of True Connection

1 Dean Ornish, *Love & Survival: 8 Pathways to Intimacy and Health* (New York: HarperCollins, 1998), xvi.

2 John Robbins, *The Food Revolution: How Your Diet Can Help Save Your Life and Our World* (San Francisco: Conari Press, 2001).

3 Parts of my personal story and some other information from this chapter were shared in my blog post: Angela Crawford, "The Power of True Connection," September 7, 2023, https://angelacrawfordphd.com/2023/09/07/the-power-of-true-connection/.

4 Roy F. Baumeister and Mark R. Leary, "The Need to Belong: Desire for Interpersonal Attachments as a Fundamental Human Motivation," *Psychological Bulletin* 117, no. 3 (1995): 497–529. https://doi.org/10.1037/0033-2909.117.3.497.

5 "Welcome to the Harvard Study of Adult Development," Harvard Second Generation Study, accessed 1/24/2024, https://www.adultdevelopmentstudy.org/.

6 Robert Waldinger, "What Makes a Good Life? Lessons from the Longest Study

on Happiness," TEDx Beacon Street, November 2015, https://www.ted.com/talks/robert_waldinger_what_makes_a_good_life_lessons_from_the_longest_study_on_happiness?language=en.

7 Waldinger, "What Makes a Good Life?" TEDx Beacon Street.

8 Ning Xia and Huige Li, "Loneliness, Social Isolation, and Cardiovascular Health," *Antioxidants & Redox Signaling* 28, no. 9 (March 20, 2018): 837–51, https://doi.org/10.1089/ars.2017.7312.

9 "Loneliness and Social Isolation Linked to Serious Health Conditions," Centers for Disease Control and Prevention, accessed January 24, 2024, https://www.cdc.gov/aging/publications/features/lonely-older-adults.html.

10 Dean Ornish, *Dr. Dean Ornish's Program for Reversing Heart Disease* (New York: Ballantine Books, 1995).

11 Ornish, *Love & Survival*, 2.

12 Ethan Kross et al., "Social Rejection Shares Somatosensory Representations with Physical Pain," *Proc Natl Acad Sci USA* 108, no. 15 (April 12, 2011): 6270–5, https://doi.org/10.1073/pnas.1102693108; Naomi I. Eisenberger, "The Neural Bases of Social Pain: Evidence for Shared Representations with Physical Pain," *Psychosom Med*, 74, no. 2 (February–March 2012): 126–35, https://doi.org/10.1097/PSY.0b013e3182464dd1.

13 Scott Barry Kaufman, *Transcend: The New Science of Self-Actualization* (New York: Penguin Random House, 2021), 38.

14 For more insight on the characteristics of healthy relationships, see Melanie Joy, *Getting Relationships Right: How to Build Resilience and Thrive in Life and Work* (Oakland, CA: Berrett-Koehler Publishers, 2020).

15 Kaufman, *Transcend*, 42; Jane Dutton and Monica Worline, "Four Ways to Create High-Quality Connections at Work," *Greater Good Magazine*, October 24, 2023, https://greatergood.berkeley.edu/article/item/four_ways_to_create_high_quality_connections_at_work.

16 Dan Buettner, *The Blue Zones: Lessons for Living Longer from the People Who've Lived the Longest* (Washington D.C.: National Geographic, 2008), 256–8.

17 Kendra Cherry, "How Social Support Contributes to Psychological Health," Very Well Mind, March 3, 2023, https://www.verywellmind.com/social-support-for-psychological-health-4119970.

18 Carol Glasser, "Veg'n Recidivism: Why Is It Happening?", Faunalytics, February 25, 2012, https://faunalytics.org/vegn-recidivism-why-is-it-happening/.

19 Rekha Sharma, "Exploring the Factors Behind Vegan Dietary Lapses," Faunalytics, June 5, 2023, https://faunalytics.org/exploring-the-factors-behind-vegan-dietary-lapses/.

20 Melanie Joy, *Beyond Beliefs: A Guide to Improving Relationships and Communication for Vegans, Vegetarians, and Meat Eaters* (New York: Lantern Books, 2018), 190–2.

21 Michael Greger, with Gene Stone, *How Not to Die* (New York: Flatiron Books, 2015), 272–5.

22 To learn more about "window cows," also called "fistulated cows" see these posts: Angela Henderson, "Why Do These Cows Have Holes Drilled into Their Sides?" PETA, last updated November 30, 2022, https://www.peta.org/blog/fistulated-cannulated-cows/; Oli Gross, "Cows Stomachs Fitted with Windows at Europe's Largest Animal Testing Centre," Totally Vegan Buzz, June 27, 2019, https://www.totallyveganbuzz.com/news/cows-stomachs-fitted-with-windows-at-europes-largest-animal-testing-centre/.

Chapter 7: Take Charge of Your Health

1 "NHE Fact Sheet," Centers for Medicare and Medicaid Services, accessed January 25, 2024, https://www.cms.gov/data-research/statistics-trends-and-reports/national-health-expenditure-data/nhe-fact-sheet.

2 Matthew McGough et al., "How Does Health Care Spending in the U.S. Compare to Other Countries?", Peterson-KFF Health System Tracker, February 9, 2023, https://www.healthsystemtracker.org/chart-collection/health-spending-u-s-compare-countries/.

3 "Life Expectancy at Birth, Total Years, All Countries and Economies," The World Bank Data, accessed January 22, 2024, https://data.worldbank.org/indicator/SP.DYN.LE00.IN.

4 "Health and Economic Costs of Chronic Diseases," Centers for Disease Control and Prevention, accessed January 25, 2024, https://www.cdc.gov/chronicdisease/about/costs/index.htm.

5 "Deaths and Mortality," Centers for Disease Control and Prevention, National Center for Health Statistics, accessed January 25, 2024, https://www.cdc.gov/nchs/fastats/deaths.htm.

6 Sari Harrar, "America's War Against Heart Disease," AARP, January 17, 2023, https://www.aarp.org/health/conditions-treatments/info-2023/fighting-heart-disease-in-america.html.

7 William F. Enos, Robert H. Holmes, and James Beyer, "Coronary Disease Among United States Soldiers Killed in Action in Korea: Preliminary Report," *JAMA* 152, no. 12 (1953): 1090–3, https://doi.org/10.1001/jama.1953.03690120006002.

8 T. Colin Campbell and Thomas M. Campbell, *The China Study* (Dallas, TX: BenBella Books, 2006), 75–6.

9 Michael Greger, *How Not to Die* (New York: Flatiron Books, 2015), 5.

10 Greger, *How Not to Die*, 6; also see graphic depicting this information: "U.S. Food Consumption as a % of Calories," Coalition for Healthy School Food, Why Change School Food?, accessed January 25, 2024, https://healthyschoolfood.org/wp/learn-more/why-change-school-food/.

11   Dan Buettner, *The Blue Zones: Lessons for Living Longer from the People Who've Lived the Longest* (Washington D.C.: National Geographic, 2008).

12   Greger, *How Not to Die*; Campbell, *The China Study*.

13   Campbell, *The China Study*, 116.

14   Campbell, *The China Study*.

15   Note: Nutrition and lifestyle are not emphasized in most medical training. Medical students receive (on average) about eleven hours of nutrition education across their entire medical education, so unless this is an area of interest for which they have sought further training, they too may be unaware of the research on plant-based nutrition. Fortunately, some medical training programs are taking steps to include more nutrition education: Elizabeth Millard, "How Nutrition Education for Doctors Is Evolving," *Time*, May 24, 2023, https://time.com/6282404/nutrition-education-doctors/.

16   Dean Ornish and Anne Ornish, *Undo It: How Simple Lifestyle Change Can Reverse Most Chronic Diseases* (New York: Ballantine Books, 2019).

17   Caldwell Esselstyn, *Prevent and Reverse Heart Disease: The Revolutionary, Scientifically Proven, Nutrition-Based Cure* (New York: Penguin Group, 2007).

18   Joel Fuhrman, "G-BOMBS: The Anti-Cancer Foods That Should Be in Your Diet Right Now," *A Doctor's Perspective* (blog), Dr. Fuhrman, July 5, 2022, https://www.drfuhrman.com/blog/237/g-bombs-the-anti-cancer-foods-that-should-be-in-your-diet-right-now.

19   Joel Fuhrman, *Eat for Life: The Breakthrough Nutrient-Rich Program for Longevity, Disease Reversal, and Sustained Weight Loss* (New York: HarperOne, 2020).

20   Neal Barnard, *Dr. Neal Barnard's Program for Reversing Diabetes* (New York: Rodale, 2017).

21   Neal Barnard, *Your Body in Balance: The New Science of Food, Hormones, and Health* (New York: Hachette Book Group, 2020); Hana Kahleova et al., "A Dietary Intervention for Postmenopausal Hot Flashes: A Potential Role of Gut Microbiome. An Exploratory Analysis," *Complement Ther Med* 79 (December 2023). https://doi.org/10.1016/j.ctim.2023.103002, https://pubmed.ncbi.nlm.nih.gov/37949415/.

22   Neal Barnard, *The Cheese Trap: How Breaking a Surprising Addiction Will Help You Lose Weight, Gain Energy, and Get Healthy* (New York: Hachette Book Group, 2017); Neal Barnard, *Power Foods For the Brain: An Effective 3-Step Plan to Protect Your Mind and Strengthen Your Memory* (New York: Grand Central Publishing, 2013).

23   Brooke Goldner, *Goodbye Lupus: How a Medical Doctor Healed Herself Naturally with Supermarket Foods* (Austin, TX: Express Results, 2015), 21.

24   Brooke Goldner, *Goodbye Lupus*; Brooke Goldner, *Goodbye Autoimmune Disease: How to Prevent and Reverse Chronic Illness and Inflammatory Symptoms Using Supermarket Foods* (Austin, TX: Express Results, 2019).

25   Mark Huberman, "Interview with Kristi Funk, M.D." *Health Science: A Publication*

of the National Health Association; Fall 2022, 5–11.

26 Dean Sherzai and Ayesha Sherzai, *The Alzheimer's Solution* (New York: HarperCollins, 2017), 3–4, 39–59.

27 To learn more about Michael Greger's books and research: Dr. Greger's books, NutritionFacts.org, https://nutritionfacts.org/books/.

28 To learn more about ultra-processed foods: Michael Greger, "Ultra-Processed Junk Food Put to the Test," NutritionFacts.org, April 25, 2022, https://nutritionfacts.org/video/ultra-processed-junk-food-put-to-the-test/.

29 As a side note, I would like to clarify that processed foods that are vegan (free of animal products) are still *much* kinder to animals and the planet, and in many cases better for human health, than animal-based alternatives. Oreos, Wonder Bread, Coke, and most potato chips happen to be technically vegan, i.e., free of animal products, but clearly wouldn't be considered health foods. However, some commercial vegan foods may be healthier than their meat-based counterparts. For example, the plant-based Beyond Burger, made from pea, rice, and fava bean proteins, has no cholesterol, 35 percent less fat, fewer calories, and none of the hormones or antibiotics found in animal-based hamburgers (information from "Cutting Through the Noise: Facts About the Health of Our Products," Beyond Meat, https://www.beyondmeat.com/en-US/whats-new/cutting-through-the-noise-facts-about-the-health-of-our-products). Dr. Michael Greger lends helpful insight regarding the nutritional comparison of animal-based and plant-based burgers in this video: Michael Greger, "Are Beyond Meat and the Impossible Burger Healthy?" NutritionFacts.org, January 19, 2024, https://nutritionfacts.org/video/friday-favorites-are-beyond-meat-and-the-impossible-burger-healthy/.

30 For those who believe that plant-based burgers are more "processed" and animal meat is more "natural," I would encourage them to take a closer look at the unhealthy conditions in which most farmed animals are raised, the unnatural diet that most are fed, the antibiotics and hormones these animals are given, the high-speed pace of slaughter, the contamination caused by the animal's intestinal contents during the slaughter process, and the intensive "processing" needed in order to bring that seemingly sanitized package of animal flesh to the grocery store. In addition, many public health issues, such as pandemics, antibiotic resistance, and foodborne illness, are directly related to animal agriculture. We would reduce many of these problems if we chose more plant-based foods, processed or not. FoodRevolution.org offers a helpful review on some of these issues: Tia Schwab, "Unhealthy Conditions for Animals Are—No Surprise—Bad for Humans, Too," Food Revolution Network (blog), March 17, 2021, https://foodrevolution.org/blog/farm-animal-cruelty-public-health/.

31 To learn more about American College of Lifestyle Medicine (ACLM), or to find a lifestyle medicine provider, visit their website: https://lifestylemedicine.org/.

32 *The Game Changers*, https://gamechangersmovie.com/.

33 Matt Frazier and Robert Cheeke, *The Plant-Based Athlete: A Game-Changing Approach to Peak Performance* (New York: HarperCollins, 2021).

34 Rich Roll, *Finding Ultra: Rejecting Middle Age, Becoming One of the Fittest Men, and Discovering Myself* (New York: Harmony Books, 2018).

35 To learn more about Chef AJ and the SOFAS-free dietary approach, visit her website: https://www.chefaj.com/.

36 For listings of plant-based or lifestyle-oriented medical providers, visit the websites of the American College of Lifestyle Medicine (https://www.lifestylemedpros. org/home), Plantrician.org (https://plantrician.org/), LoveLife Telehealth (https://love.life/telehealth/find-your-doctor/), or Physicians Committee for Responsible Medicine (https://www.pcrm.org/findadoctor/search-telehealth).

Chapter 8: Discover Your Interconnectedness with Life

1 William James, *The Varieties of Religious Experience* (Cambridge, MA: Harvard University Press, 1902).

2 "Spirituality," *Psychology Today*, accessed 1/25/2024, https://www. psychologytoday.com/us/basics/spirituality.

3 Timothy B. Smith et al., "Religiousness and Depression: Evidence for a Main Effect and the Moderating Influence of Stressful Life Events," *Psychol Bull* 129, no. 4 (July 2003): 614–36, https://doi.org/10.1037/0033-2909.129.4.614.

4 Lisa Miller, *The Awakened Brain: The Psychology of Spirituality* (New York: Penguin Books, 2021), 8.

5 Miller, *The Awakened Brain*, 7–8.

6 Miller, *The Awakened Brain*, 7.

7 Miller, *The Awakened Brain*, 163.

8 Miller, *The Awakened Brain*, 164–6.

9 Daniel Siegel, *Mindsight: The New Science of Personal Transformation* (New York: Bantam Books, 2010).

10 Scott Barry Kaufman, *Transcend: The New Science of Self-Actualization* (New York: Penguin Random House, 2020), 218.

11 David Bryce Yaden et al., "The Varieties of Self-Transcendent Experience," *Review of General Psychology* 21, no. 2 (2017): 143–60, https://doi.org/10.1037/ gpr0000102.

12 Kaufman, *Transcend*, 202.

13 Kaufman, *Transcend*, 203.

14 Kaufman, *Transcend*, 220.

15 Kaufman, *Transcend*, 223

16 Kelly Miller, "Science of Spirituality (+ 16 Ways to Become More Spiritual)," Positive Psychology, April 16, 2020, https://positivepsychology.com/science- of-spirituality/.

17 There are numerous sources on veganism and spirituality, some of which are listed in the Resources section at the back of this book. The documentary *A Prayer for Compassion* (http://aprayerforcompassion.com/) addresses this connection in depth.

18 Victoria Moran, "Why Vegan Spirituality Matters," *Main Street Vegan Academy* (blog), September 5, 2023, https://mainstreetvegan.com/why-vegan-spirituality-matters-by-victoria-moran-chc-mvlce-ryt-200/.

19 The Daniel Fast is utilized in many Christian churches as a way to clean up one's diet and connect more deeply with God, based on the book of Daniel. If you are interested in learning more, here is some recommended reading: Sersie Blue and Gigi Carter, *The Daniel Fast: Why You Should Only Do it Once* (Tustin, CA: Trilogy Christian Publishers, 2023).

20 Lisa Kemmerer, *Vegan Ethics: AMORE—Five Reasons to Choose Vegan* (Vegan Tapestry, 2002), 47–85.

21 Carol J. Adams, *The Inner Art of Vegetarianism: Spiritual Practices for Body and Soul* (New York: Lantern Books, 2000), 9–11.

22 For a discussion on how the suffering and stress of animals in factory farms may be passed on to those of us who consume them: Lani Muelrath, *The Mindful Vegan: A 30-Day Plan for Finding Health, Balance, Peace, and Happiness* (Dallas, TX: BenBella Books, 2017), Day Seventeen, Moods and Foods (locator 2572, Kindle edition).

23 Will Tuttle, Ph.D., *The World Peace Diet: Eating for Spiritual Health and Social Harmony, 10th anniversary ed.* (New York: Lantern Books, 2016), 135.

24 Tuttle, *The World Peace Diet*; Hope Ferdowsian, *The Phoenix Zones: Where Strength Is Born and Resilience Lives* (Chicago: University of Chicago Press, 2018); Melanie Joy, *How to End Injustice Everywhere: Understanding the Common Denominator Driving All Injustices, to Create a Better World for Humans, Animals, and the Planet* (New York: Lantern Publishing & Media, 2023).

25 Ferdowsian, *The Phoenix Zones*, 32.

26 *The Holy Bible*, New International Version (Grand Rapids, MI: Zondervan Publishing House, 1984), Ecclesiastes 1:18: "For with much wisdom comes much sorrow; the more knowledge, the more grief."

27 There are many helpful books, websites, and apps to support you with meditation practice. Some apps to consider: Headspace, https://www.headspace.com/; Insight Timer, https://insighttimer.com/; and the JKZ Meditation app (by Jon Kabat-Zinn), https://jonkabat-zinn.com/meditation-app/. In addition, Tara Brach, Ph.D. offers many helpful meditation resources on her website, https://www.tarabrach.com/.

28 My audio recording of this exercise is available at: https://angelacrawfordphd.com/meditations/.

Chapter 9: Keys to Successful Lifestyle Change

1 James O. Prochaska and Janice M. Prochaska, *Changing to Thrive: Using the Stages of Change to Overcome the Top Threats to Your Health and Happiness* (Center City: MN: Hazelden Publishing, 2016), xiii.

2 James Clear, *Atomic Habits: An Easy and Proven Way to Build Good Habits & Break Bad Ones* (New York: Penguin Random House, 2018), 34.

3 B.J. Fogg, *Tiny Habits: The Small Changes that Change Everything* (New York: First Mariner Books, 2020), 2.

4 Some self-help books on behavior and lifestyle change that I have found helpful: Clear, *Atomic Habits*; Fogg, *Tiny Habits*; Prochaska and Prochaska, *Change to Thrive*; and Gary Foster, *The Shift: 7 Powerful Mindset Changes for Lasting Weight Loss* (New York: St. Martin's Griffin, 2021).

5 The "SMART" goals concept is widely used in literature on goal setting. Reportedly, it first appeared in a November 1981 issue of *Management Review* (vol. 70, no. 11), in an article titled, "There's a S.M.A.R.T. Way to Write Management's Goals and Objectives," by George Doran, Arthur Miller, and James Cunningham.

6 When I say that we all have different "parts," I am not referring to dissociative identity disorder (formerly known as multiple personality disorder), a psychiatric disorder that stems from severe trauma. Study of "normal" psychology suggests that we are all made up of different ego states, which may serve a variety of roles and/or have differing feelings or motivations. Most of us have some awareness of these differing parts, even though we may not give this much thought in daily life. Working with inner parts is an effective (and self-compassionate) way to work through inner conflicts and blocks. To learn more about the concept of internal parts, check out books on Internal Family Systems (IFS), such as *Introduction to Internal Family Systems* by Richard Schwartz, Ph.D.; *No Bad Parts* by Richard Schwartz, Ph.D.; or *Self-Therapy* by Jay Earley, Ph.D.

7 Dan Buettner, *The Blue Zones: Lessons for Living Longer from the People Who've Lived the Longest* (Washington D.C.: National Geographic, 2008).

8 Behavior change can be complex, and when we try to push others to change, it is human nature for them to resist. People are generally more motivated to change when they come to an inner sense that it is the right or best choice for them (rather than feeling pressured by another person). I recommend the book *Beyond Beliefs: A Guide to Improving Relationships and Communication for Vegans, Vegetarians, and Meat Eaters* by Melanie Joy, Ph.D., to gain insights and skills for effective communication approaches.

9 Research by Faunalytics found that vegetarians and vegans who maintained a veg lifestyle often had multiple motivating reasons, including not only

personal health but also ethical and/or environmental considerations. See: "Study of Current and Former Vegetarians and Vegans: Initial Findings," Humane Research Council (HRC), December 2014, https://faunalytics.org/wp-content/uploads/2015/06/Faunalytics_Current-Former-Vegetarians_Full-Report.pdf; "A Summary of Faunalytics' Study of Current and Former Vegetarians and Vegans," Faunalytics, February 24, 2016, https://faunalytics.org/a-summary-of-faunalytics-study-of-current-and-former-vegetarians-and-vegans/.

Chapter 10: Thriving Emotionally and Socially as a Vegan

1   Melanie Joy, *Beyond Beliefs: A Guide to Improving Relationships and Communication for Vegans, Vegetarians, and Meat Eaters* (New York: Lantern Books, 2018), 5.

2   Clare Mann, *Vystopia: The Anguish of Being Vegan in a Non-Vegan World* (Sydney Australia: Communicate31, 2018), 30–45.

3   Mann, *Vystopia*, 43 (my italics).

4   Gabor Maté with Daniel Maté, *The Myth of Normal: Trauma, Illness & Healing in a Toxic Culture* (New York: Avery, 2022), 19–20.

5   American Psychiatric Association, *Diagnostic and Statistical Manual of Mental Disorders, 5th ed.: DSM-V* (Arlington, VA: American Psychiatric Publishing, 2013). Note: The DSM-V considers someone to meet criteria for Post-Traumatic Stress Disorder (PTSD) if they were exposed to a traumatic event and subsequently experience various trauma-related symptoms (intrusion symptoms, avoidance symptoms, cognitive and mood disturbance, and alterations in arousal and reactivity) lasting more than one month and causing clinically significant distress or impairment. DSM-V has expanded their definition of exposure to a traumatic event (compared to earlier versions of the manual) to include not only those who are direct victims of violence, but also those who witness, learn about, or have repeated or extreme exposure to details of trauma or violence happening to others (vicarious or secondary trauma).

6   See Joy, *Beyond Beliefs*, for an excellent discussion of Secondary Traumatic Stress (STS) and its symptoms and impacts as applied to vegans, 99–100, 203.

7   For example, Dr. Melanie Joy, Clare Mann, and Colleen Patrick-Goudreau, along with other authors listed in the Resources for Thriving Emotionally and Socially in the back of this book.

8   Victor E. Frankl, *Man's Search for Meaning* (Boston, MA: Beacon Press, 1959), 76.

9   Melanie Joy, *Why We Love Dogs, Eat Pigs, and Wear Cows: An Introduction to Carnism* (San Francisco, CA: Conari Press, 2010).

10 Happy Cow website: https://www.happycow.net/.

11 Kerry Patterson et al., *Crucial Conversations: Tools for Talking When the Stakes Are High* (New York: McGraw-Hill, 2012), 33–49.

12 To learn more about assertive communication, here is a good summary article: Elizabeth Scott, "How to Use Assertive Communication," Very Well Mind, updated September 26, 2023, https://www.verywellmind.com/learn-assertive-communication-in-five-simple-steps-3144969. For more in-depth information about communication skills, see Matthew McKay, Martha Davis, and Patrick Fanning, *Messages: The Communication Skills Book* (Oakland, CA: New Harbinger, 2018).

13 Patterson et al., *Crucial Conversations*.

14 For example, *Crucial Conversations*; *Beyond Beliefs*; *Messages: The Communication Skills Book*; or other books listed in the Resources section.

15 Psychologist Tara Brach, Ph.D., has helpful resources for mindfulness on her website: https://www.tarabrach.com/.

16 Books I have found helpful include Elaine Aron, *The Highly Sensitive Person: How to Thrive When the World Overwhelms You* (New York: Citadel Press, 1996); Judith Orloff, *The Empath's Survival Guide: Life Strategies for Sensitive People* (Boulder, CO: Sounds True, 2017).

17 In Defense of Animals (IDA) has a list of psychotherapists who are sensitive to vegan and animal activist issues: https://www.idausa.org/campaign/sustainable-activism/activist-resource-list/#therapistAA. For those who are experiencing significant trauma symptoms, a highly effective therapeutic approach is Eye Movement Desensitization and Reprocessing (EMDR). You can locate psychotherapists trained in this approach on the EMDR International Association (EMDRIA) website: https://www.emdria.org/find-an-emdr-therapist/.

18 An audio recording of a meditation for Visualizing a Vegan World is available on my website: https://angelacrawfordphd.com/meditations/.

19 To learn more about Rae Sikora, see her essay, "There Is No Other," in *Vegan Voices: Essays by Inspiring Changemakers* (Joanne Kong, ed., New York: Lantern, 2021), 36–9.

11: Moving Toward a Compassionate World

1 Victoria Moran, with Adair Moran, *Main Street Vegan: Everything You Need to Know to Eat Healthfully and Live Compassionately in the Real World* (New York: Penguin, 2012), 343.

2 Tara Brach, *Radical Compassion: Learning to Love Yourself and Your World with the Practice of RAIN* (New York: Penguin Random House, 2019), xvii.

ABOUT THE AUTHOR

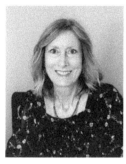 With twenty-five years of experience as a clinical psychologist, Angela Crawford, Ph.D., is passionate about sharing the benefits of a plant-powered, vegan lifestyle for emotional, mental, spiritual, and physical health. She writes, teaches, and speaks about thriving with a plant-based lifestyle, living compassionately, and discovering greater well-being and purpose.

Dr. Crawford previously worked as a psychotherapist for over two decades, empowering clients to make lifestyle changes to address stress and trauma and achieve holistic well-being. She holds certificates in plant-based nutrition, as a master vegan lifestyle coach and educator, as a transformational coach, and as an EMDR practitioner. She lives with her husband in upstate New York. You can learn more about Dr. Crawford's work through her website: angelacrawfordphd.com.

ABOUT THE PUBLISHER

Lantern Publishing & Media was founded in 2020 to follow and expand on the legacy of Lantern Books—a publishing company started in 1999 on the principles of living with a greater depth and commitment to the preservation of the natural world. Like its predecessor, Lantern Publishing & Media produces books on animal advocacy, veganism, religion, social justice, humane education, psychology, family therapy, and recovery. Lantern is dedicated to printing in the United States on recycled paper and saving resources in our day-to-day operations. Our titles are also available as ebooks and audiobooks.

To catch up on Lantern's publishing program, visit us at www.lanternpm.org.

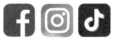 facebook.com/lanternpm
instagram.com/lanternpm
tiktok.com/@lanternpmofficial